CCTN
Exam

SECRETS

Study Guide
Your Key to Exam Success

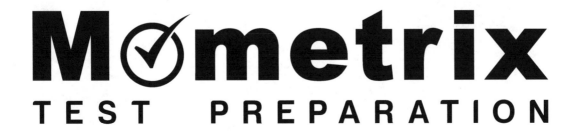

DEAR FUTURE EXAM SUCCESS STORY

First of all, **THANK YOU** for purchasing Mometrix study materials!

Second, congratulations! You are one of the few determined test-takers who are committed to doing whatever it takes to excel on your exam. **You have come to the right place.** We developed these study materials with one goal in mind: to deliver you the information you need in a format that's concise and easy to use.

In addition to optimizing your guide for the content of the test, we've outlined our recommended steps for breaking down the preparation process into small, attainable goals so you can make sure you stay on track.

We've also analyzed the entire test-taking process, identifying the most common pitfalls and showing how you can overcome them and be ready for any curveball the test throws you.

Standardized testing is one of the biggest obstacles on your road to success, which only increases the importance of doing well in the high-pressure, high-stakes environment of test day. Your results on this test could have a significant impact on your future, and this guide provides the information and practical advice to help you achieve your full potential on test day.

Your success is our success

We would love to hear from you! If you would like to share the story of your exam success or if you have any questions or comments in regard to our products, please contact us at **800-673-8175** or **support@mometrix.com**.

Thanks again for your business and we wish you continued success!

Sincerely,
The Mometrix Test Preparation Team

Need more help? Check out our flashcards at:
http://mometrixflashcards.com/CCTN

TABLE OF CONTENTS

Introduction

Thank you for purchasing this resource! You have made the choice to prepare yourself for a test that could have a huge impact on your future, and this guide is designed to help you be fully ready for test day. Obviously, it's important to have a solid understanding of the test material, but you also need to be prepared for the unique environment and stressors of the test, so that you can perform to the best of your abilities.

For this purpose, the first section that appears in this guide is the **Secret Keys**. We've devoted countless hours to meticulously researching what works and what doesn't, and we've boiled down our findings to the five most impactful steps you can take to improve your performance on the test. We start at the beginning with study planning and move through the preparation process, all the way to the testing strategies that will help you get the most out of what you know when you're finally sitting in front of the test.

We recommend that you start preparing for your test as far in advance as possible. However, if you've bought this guide as a last-minute study resource and only have a few days before your test, we recommend that you skip over the first two Secret Keys since they address a long-term study plan.

If you struggle with **test anxiety**, we strongly encourage you to check out our recommendations for how you can overcome it. Test anxiety is a formidable foe, but it can be beaten, and we want to make sure you have the tools you need to defeat it.

1

Secret Key #1 – Plan Big, Study Small

There's a lot riding on your performance. If you want to ace this test, you're going to need to keep your skills sharp and the material fresh in your mind. You need a plan that lets you review everything you need to know while still fitting in your schedule. We'll break this strategy down into three categories.

Information Organization

Start with the information you already have: the official test outline. From this, you can make a complete list of all the concepts you need to cover before the test. Organize these concepts into groups that can be studied together, and create a list of any related vocabulary you need to learn so you can brush up on any difficult terms. You'll want to keep this vocabulary list handy once you actually start studying since you may need to add to it along the way.

Time Management

Once you have your set of study concepts, decide how to spread them out over the time you have left before the test. Break your study plan into small, clear goals so you have a manageable task for each day and know exactly what you're doing. Then just focus on one small step at a time. When you manage your time this way, you don't need to spend hours at a time studying. Studying a small block of content for a short period each day helps you retain information better and avoid stressing over how much you have left to do. You can relax knowing that you have a plan to cover everything in time. In order for this strategy to be effective though, you have to start studying early and stick to your schedule. Avoid the exhaustion and futility that comes from last-minute cramming!

Study Environment

The environment you study in has a big impact on your learning. Studying in a coffee shop, while probably more enjoyable, is not likely to be as fruitful as studying in a quiet room. It's important to keep distractions to a minimum. You're only planning to study for a short block of time, so make the most of it. Don't pause to check your phone or get up to find a snack. It's also important to **avoid multitasking**. Research has consistently shown that multitasking will make your studying dramatically less effective. Your study area should also be comfortable and well-lit so you don't have the distraction of straining your eyes or sitting on an uncomfortable chair.

The time of day you study is also important. You want to be rested and alert. Don't wait until just before bedtime. Study when you'll be most likely to comprehend and remember. Even better, if you know what time of day your test will be, set that time aside for study. That way your brain will be used to working on that subject at that specific time and you'll have a better chance of recalling information.

Finally, it can be helpful to team up with others who are studying for the same test. Your actual studying should be done in as isolated an environment as possible, but the work of organizing the information and setting up the study plan can be divided up. In between study sessions, you can discuss with your teammates the concepts that you're all studying and quiz each other on the details. Just be sure that your teammates are as serious about the test as you are. If you find that your study time is being replaced with social time, you might need to find a new team.

Secret Key #2 – Make Your Studying Count

You're devoting a lot of time and effort to preparing for this test, so you want to be absolutely certain it will pay off. This means doing more than just reading the content and hoping you can remember it on test day. It's important to make every minute of study count. There are two main areas you can focus on to make your studying count:

Retention

It doesn't matter how much time you study if you can't remember the material. You need to make sure you are retaining the concepts. To check your retention of the information you're learning, try recalling it at later times with minimal prompting. Try carrying around flashcards and glance at one or two from time to time or ask a friend who's also studying for the test to quiz you.

To enhance your retention, look for ways to put the information into practice so that you can apply it rather than simply recalling it. If you're using the information in practical ways, it will be much easier to remember. Similarly, it helps to solidify a concept in your mind if you're not only reading it to yourself but also explaining it to someone else. Ask a friend to let you teach them about a concept you're a little shaky on (or speak aloud to an imaginary audience if necessary). As you try to summarize, define, give examples, and answer your friend's questions, you'll understand the concepts better and they will stay with you longer. Finally, step back for a big picture view and ask yourself how each piece of information fits with the whole subject. When you link the different concepts together and see them working together as a whole, it's easier to remember the individual components.

Finally, practice showing your work on any multi-step problems, even if you're just studying. Writing out each step you take to solve a problem will help solidify the process in your mind, and you'll be more likely to remember it during the test.

Modality

Modality simply refers to the means or method by which you study. Choosing a study modality that fits your own individual learning style is crucial. No two people learn best in exactly the same way, so it's important to know your strengths and use them to your advantage.

For example, if you learn best by visualization, focus on visualizing a concept in your mind and draw an image or a diagram. Try color-coding your notes, illustrating them, or creating symbols that will trigger your mind to recall a learned concept. If you learn best by hearing or discussing information, find a study partner who learns the same way or read aloud to yourself. Think about how to put the information in your own words. Imagine that you are giving a lecture on the topic and record yourself so you can listen to it later.

For any learning style, flashcards can be helpful. Organize the information so you can take advantage of spare moments to review. Underline key words or phrases. Use different colors for different categories. Mnemonic devices (such as creating a short list in which every item starts with the same letter) can also help with retention. Find what works best for you and use it to store the information in your mind most effectively and easily.

3

Secret Key #3 – Practice the Right Way

Your success on test day depends not only on how many hours you put into preparing, but also on whether you prepared the right way. It's good to check along the way to see if your studying is paying off. One of the most effective ways to do this is by taking practice tests to evaluate your progress. Practice tests are useful because they show exactly where you need to improve. Every time you take a practice test, pay special attention to these three groups of questions:

- The questions you got wrong
- The questions you had to guess on, even if you guessed right
- The questions you found difficult or slow to work through

This will show you exactly what your weak areas are, and where you need to devote more study time. Ask yourself why each of these questions gave you trouble. Was it because you didn't understand the material? Was it because you didn't remember the vocabulary? Do you need more repetitions on this type of question to build speed and confidence? Dig into those questions and figure out how you can strengthen your weak areas as you go back to review the material.

Additionally, many practice tests have a section explaining the answer choices. It can be tempting to read the explanation and think that you now have a good understanding of the concept. However, an explanation likely only covers part of the question's broader context. Even if the explanation makes sense, **go back and investigate** every concept related to the question until you're positive you have a thorough understanding.

As you go along, keep in mind that the practice test is just that: practice. Memorizing these questions and answers will not be very helpful on the actual test because it is unlikely to have any of the same exact questions. If you only know the right answers to the sample questions, you won't be prepared for the real thing. **Study the concepts** until you understand them fully, and then you'll be able to answer any question that shows up on the test.

It's important to wait on the practice tests until you're ready. If you take a test on your first day of study, you may be overwhelmed by the amount of material covered and how much you need to learn. Work up to it gradually.

On test day, you'll need to be prepared for answering questions, managing your time, and using the test-taking strategies you've learned. It's a lot to balance, like a mental marathon that will have a big impact on your future. Like training for a marathon, you'll need to start slowly and work your way up. When test day arrives, you'll be ready.

Start with the strategies you've read in the first two Secret Keys—plan your course and study in the way that works best for you. If you have time, consider using multiple study resources to get different approaches to the same concepts. It can be helpful to see difficult concepts from more than one angle. Then find a good source for practice tests. Many times, the test website will suggest potential study resources or provide sample tests.

Practice Test Strategy

If you're able to find at least three practice tests, we recommend this strategy:

UNTIMED AND OPEN-BOOK PRACTICE

Take the first test with no time constraints and with your notes and study guide handy. Take your time and focus on applying the strategies you've learned.

TIMED AND OPEN-BOOK PRACTICE

Take the second practice test open-book as well, but set a timer and practice pacing yourself to finish in time.

TIMED AND CLOSED-BOOK PRACTICE

Take any other practice tests as if it were test day. Set a timer and put away your study materials. Sit at a table or desk in a quiet room, imagine yourself at the testing center, and answer questions as quickly and accurately as possible.

Keep repeating timed and closed-book tests on a regular basis until you run out of practice tests or it's time for the actual test. Your mind will be ready for the schedule and stress of test day, and you'll be able to focus on recalling the material you've learned.

Secret Key #4 – Pace Yourself

Once you're fully prepared for the material on the test, your biggest challenge on test day will be managing your time. Just knowing that the clock is ticking can make you panic even if you have plenty of time left. Work on pacing yourself so you can build confidence against the time constraints of the exam. Pacing is a difficult skill to master, especially in a high-pressure environment, so **practice is vital**.

Set time expectations for your pace based on how much time is available. For example, if a section has 60 questions and the time limit is 30 minutes, you know you have to average 30 seconds or less per question in order to answer them all. Although 30 seconds is the hard limit, set 25 seconds per question as your goal, so you reserve extra time to spend on harder questions. When you budget extra time for the harder questions, you no longer have any reason to stress when those questions take longer to answer.

Don't let this time expectation distract you from working through the test at a calm, steady pace, but keep it in mind so you don't spend too much time on any one question. Recognize that taking extra time on one question you don't understand may keep you from answering two that you do understand later in the test. If your time limit for a question is up and you're still not sure of the answer, mark it and move on, and come back to it later if the time and the test format allow. If the testing format doesn't allow you to return to earlier questions, just make an educated guess; then put it out of your mind and move on.

On the easier questions, be careful not to rush. It may seem wise to hurry through them so you have more time for the challenging ones, but it's not worth missing one if you know the concept and just didn't take the time to read the question fully. Work efficiently but make sure you understand the question and have looked at all of the answer choices, since more than one may seem right at first.

Even if you're paying attention to the time, you may find yourself a little behind at some point. You should speed up to get back on track, but do so wisely. Don't panic; just take a few seconds less on each question until you're caught up. Don't guess without thinking, but do look through the answer choices and eliminate any you know are wrong. If you can get down to two choices, it is often worthwhile to guess from those. Once you've chosen an answer, move on and don't dwell on any that you skipped or had to hurry through. If a question was taking too long, chances are it was one of the harder ones, so you weren't as likely to get it right anyway.

On the other hand, if you find yourself getting ahead of schedule, it may be beneficial to slow down a little. The more quickly you work, the more likely you are to make a careless mistake that will affect your score. You've budgeted time for each question, so don't be afraid to spend that time. Practice an efficient but careful pace to get the most out of the time you have.

Secret Key #5 – Have a Plan for Guessing

When you're taking the test, you may find yourself stuck on a question. Some of the answer choices seem better than others, but you don't see the one answer choice that is obviously correct. What do you do?

The scenario described above is very common, yet most test takers have not effectively prepared for it. Developing and practicing a plan for guessing may be one of the single most effective uses of your time as you get ready for the exam.

In developing your plan for guessing, there are three questions to address:

- When should you start the guessing process?
- How should you narrow down the choices?
- Which answer should you choose?

When to Start the Guessing Process

Unless your plan for guessing is to select C every time (which, despite its merits, is not what we recommend), you need to leave yourself enough time to apply your answer elimination strategies. Since you have a limited amount of time for each question, that means that if you're going to give yourself the best shot at guessing correctly, you have to decide quickly whether or not you will guess.

Of course, the best-case scenario is that you don't have to guess at all, so first, see if you can answer the question based on your knowledge of the subject and basic reasoning skills. Focus on the key words in the question and try to jog your memory of related topics. Give yourself a chance to bring the knowledge to mind, but once you realize that you don't have (or you can't access) the knowledge you need to answer the question, it's time to start the guessing process.

It's almost always better to start the guessing process too early than too late. It only takes a few seconds to remember something and answer the question from knowledge. Carefully eliminating wrong answer choices takes longer. Plus, going through the process of eliminating answer choices can actually help jog your memory.

Summary: Start the guessing process as soon as you decide that you can't answer the question based on your knowledge.

7

How to Narrow Down the Choices

The next chapter in this book (**Test-Taking Strategies**) includes a wide range of strategies for how to approach questions and how to look for answer choices to eliminate. You will definitely want to read those carefully, practice them, and figure out which ones work best for you. Here though, we're going to address a mindset rather than a particular strategy.

Your chances of guessing an answer correctly depend on how many options you are choosing from.

How many choices you have	How likely you are to guess correctly
5	20%
4	25%
3	33%
2	50%
1	100%

You can see from this chart just how valuable it is to be able to eliminate incorrect answers and make an educated guess, but there are two things that many test takers do that cause them to miss out on the benefits of guessing:

- Accidentally eliminating the correct answer
- Selecting an answer based on an impression

We'll look at the first one here, and the second one in the next section.

To avoid accidentally eliminating the correct answer, we recommend a thought exercise called **the $5 challenge**. In this challenge, you only eliminate an answer choice from contention if you are willing to bet $5 on it being wrong. Why $5? Five dollars is a small but not insignificant amount of money. It's an amount you could afford to lose but wouldn't want to throw away. And while losing $5 once might not hurt too much, doing it twenty times will set you back $100. In the same way, each small decision you make—eliminating a choice here, guessing on a question there—won't by itself impact your score very much, but when you put them all together, they can make a big difference. By holding each answer choice elimination decision to a higher standard, you can reduce the risk of accidentally eliminating the correct answer.

The $5 challenge can also be applied in a positive sense: If you are willing to bet $5 that an answer choice *is* correct, go ahead and mark it as correct.

Summary: Only eliminate an answer choice if you are willing to bet $5 that it is wrong.

Which Answer to Choose

You're taking the test. You've run into a hard question and decided you'll have to guess. You've eliminated all the answer choices you're willing to bet $5 on. Now you have to pick an answer. Why do we even need to talk about this? Why can't you just pick whichever one you feel like when the time comes?

The answer to these questions is that if you don't come into the test with a plan, you'll rely on your impression to select an answer choice, and if you do that, you risk falling into a trap. The test writers know that everyone who takes their test will be guessing on some of the questions, so they intentionally write wrong answer choices to seem plausible. You still have to pick an answer though, and if the wrong answer choices are designed to look right, how can you ever be sure that you're not falling for their trap? The best solution we've found to this dilemma is to take the decision out of your hands entirely. Here is the process we recommend:

Once you've eliminated any choices that you are confident (willing to bet $5) are wrong, select the first remaining choice as your answer.

Whether you choose to select the first remaining choice, the second, or the last, the important thing is that you use some preselected standard. Using this approach guarantees that you will not be enticed into selecting an answer choice that looks right, because you are not basing your decision on how the answer choices look.

This is not meant to make you question your knowledge. Instead, it is to help you recognize the difference between your knowledge and your impressions. There's a huge difference between thinking an answer is right because of what you know, and thinking an answer is right because it looks or sounds like it should be right.

Summary: To ensure that your selection is appropriately random, make a predetermined selection from among all answer choices you have not eliminated.

Test-Taking Strategies

This section contains a list of test-taking strategies that you may find helpful as you work through the test. By taking what you know and applying logical thought, you can maximize your chances of answering any question correctly!

It is very important to realize that every question is different and every person is different: no single strategy will work on every question, and no single strategy will work for every person. That's why we've included all of them here, so you can try them out and determine which ones work best for different types of questions and which ones work best for you.

Question Strategies

READ CAREFULLY

Read the question and answer choices carefully. Don't miss the question because you misread the terms. You have plenty of time to read each question thoroughly and make sure you understand what is being asked. Yet a happy medium must be attained, so don't waste too much time. You must read carefully, but efficiently.

CONTEXTUAL CLUES

Look for contextual clues. If the question includes a word you are not familiar with, look at the immediate context for some indication of what the word might mean. Contextual clues can often give you all the information you need to decipher the meaning of an unfamiliar word. Even if you can't determine the meaning, you may be able to narrow down the possibilities enough to make a solid guess at the answer to the question.

PREFIXES

If you're having trouble with a word in the question or answer choices, try dissecting it. Take advantage of every clue that the word might include. Prefixes and suffixes can be a huge help. Usually they allow you to determine a basic meaning. Pre- means before, post- means after, pro - is positive, de- is negative. From prefixes and suffixes, you can get an idea of the general meaning of the word and try to put it into context.

HEDGE WORDS

Watch out for critical hedge words, such as *likely, may, can, sometimes, often, almost, mostly, usually, generally, rarely,* and *sometimes.* Question writers insert these hedge phrases to cover every possibility. Often an answer choice will be wrong simply because it leaves no room for exception. Be on guard for answer choices that have definitive words such as *exactly* and *always.*

SWITCHBACK WORDS

Stay alert for *switchbacks*. These are the words and phrases frequently used to alert you to shifts in thought. The most common switchback words are *but, although,* and *however.* Others include *nevertheless, on the other hand, even though, while, in spite of, despite, regardless of.* Switchback words are important to catch because they can change the direction of the question or an answer choice.

FACE VALUE

When in doubt, use common sense. Accept the situation in the problem at face value. Don't read too much into it. These problems will not require you to make wild assumptions. If you have to go beyond creativity and warp time or space in order to have an answer choice fit the question, then you should move on and consider the other answer choices. These are normal problems rooted in reality. The applicable relationship or explanation may not be readily apparent, but it is there for you to figure out. Use your common sense to interpret anything that isn't clear.

Answer Choice Strategies

ANSWER SELECTION

The most thorough way to pick an answer choice is to identify and eliminate wrong answers until only one is left, then confirm it is the correct answer. Sometimes an answer choice may immediately seem right, but be careful. The test writers will usually put more than one reasonable answer choice on each question, so take a second to read all of them and make sure that the other choices are not equally obvious. As long as you have time left, it is better to read every answer choice than to pick the first one that looks right without checking the others.

ANSWER CHOICE FAMILIES

An answer choice family consists of two (in rare cases, three) answer choices that are very similar in construction and cannot all be true at the same time. If you see two answer choices that are direct opposites or parallels, one of them is usually the correct answer. For instance, if one answer choice says that quantity x increases and another either says that quantity x decreases (opposite) or says that quantity y increases (parallel), then those answer choices would fall into the same family. An answer choice that doesn't match the construction of the answer choice family is more likely to be incorrect. Most questions will not have answer choice families, but when they do appear, you should be prepared to recognize them.

ELIMINATE ANSWERS

Eliminate answer choices as soon as you realize they are wrong, but make sure you consider all possibilities. If you are eliminating answer choices and realize that the last one you are left with is also wrong, don't panic. Start over and consider each choice again. There may be something you missed the first time that you will realize on the second pass.

AVOID FACT TRAPS

Don't be distracted by an answer choice that is factually true but doesn't answer the question. You are looking for the choice that answers the question. Stay focused on what the question is asking for so you don't accidentally pick an answer that is true but incorrect. Always go back to the question and make sure the answer choice you've selected actually answers the question and is not merely a true statement.

EXTREME STATEMENTS

In general, you should avoid answers that put forth extreme actions as standard practice or proclaim controversial ideas as established fact. An answer choice that states the "process should be used in certain situations, if..." is much more likely to be correct than one that states the "process should be discontinued completely." The first is a calm rational statement and doesn't even make a definitive, uncompromising stance, using a hedge word *if* to provide wiggle room, whereas the second choice is a radical idea and far more extreme.

BENCHMARK

As you read through the answer choices and you come across one that seems to answer the question well, mentally select that answer choice. This is not your final answer, but it's the one that will help you evaluate the other answer choices. The one that you selected is your benchmark or standard for judging each of the other answer choices. Every other answer choice must be compared to your benchmark. That choice is correct until proven otherwise by another answer choice beating it. If you find a better answer, then that one becomes your new benchmark. Once you've decided that no other choice answers the question as well as your benchmark, you have your final answer.

PREDICT THE ANSWER

Before you even start looking at the answer choices, it is often best to try to predict the answer. When you come up with the answer on your own, it is easier to avoid distractions and traps because you will know exactly what to look for. The right answer choice is unlikely to be word-for-word what you came up with, but it should be a close match. Even if you are confident that you have the right answer, you should still take the time to read each option before moving on.

General Strategies

TOUGH QUESTIONS

If you are stumped on a problem or it appears too hard or too difficult, don't waste time. Move on! Remember though, if you can quickly check for obviously incorrect answer choices, your chances of guessing correctly are greatly improved. Before you completely give up, at least try to knock out a couple of possible answers. Eliminate what you can and then guess at the remaining answer choices before moving on.

CHECK YOUR WORK

Since you will probably not know every term listed and the answer to every question, it is important that you get credit for the ones that you do know. Don't miss any questions through careless mistakes. If at all possible, try to take a second to look back over your answer selection and make sure you've selected the correct answer choice and haven't made a costly careless mistake (such as marking an answer choice that you didn't mean to mark). This quick double check should more than pay for itself in caught mistakes for the time it costs.

PACE YOURSELF

It's easy to be overwhelmed when you're looking at a page full of questions; your mind is confused and full of random thoughts, and the clock is ticking down faster than you would like. Calm down and maintain the pace that you have set for yourself. Especially as you get down to the last few minutes of the test, don't let the small numbers on the clock make you panic. As long as you are on track by monitoring your pace, you are guaranteed to have time for each question.

DON'T RUSH

It is very easy to make errors when you are in a hurry. Maintaining a fast pace in answering questions is pointless if it makes you miss questions that you would have gotten right otherwise. Test writers like to include distracting information and wrong answers that seem right. Taking a little extra time to avoid careless mistakes can make all the difference in your test score. Find a pace that allows you to be confident in the answers that you select.

KEEP MOVING

Panicking will not help you pass the test, so do your best to stay calm and keep moving. Taking deep breaths and going through the answer elimination steps you practiced can help to break through a stress barrier and keep your pace.

Final Notes

The combination of a solid foundation of content knowledge and the confidence that comes from practicing your plan for applying that knowledge is the key to maximizing your performance on test day. As your foundation of content knowledge is built up and strengthened, you'll find that the strategies included in this chapter become more and more effective in helping you quickly sift through the distractions and traps of the test to isolate the correct answer.

Now it's time to move on to the test content chapters of this book, but be sure to keep your goal in mind. As you read, think about how you will be able to apply this information on the test. If you've already seen sample questions for the test and you have an idea of the question format and style, try to come up with questions of your own that you can answer based on what you're reading. This will give you valuable practice applying your knowledge in the same ways you can expect to on test day.

Good luck and good studying!

General Transplantation Care

Common Diseases Requiring Transplant

COMMON DISEASES THAT REQUIRE PANCREAS OR LIVER TRANSPLANT

The most common disease that requires a **pancreas transplant** is brittle Type I diabetes (IDDM) with no signs of advanced diabetic nephropathy. Potential pancreas recipients who are not on dialysis must undergo the same tests as kidney recipients.

The most common diseases that require a **liver transplant** are:

- Alcoholism with liver changes
- Cholestasis
- Chronic hepatitis
- Genetic diseases (Crigler-Najjar syndrome, hereditary oxalosis, familial hypercholesterolemia, etc.)
- Hepatocellular carcinoma less than 5 cm accompanied by cirrhosis
- Metabolic disease

Symptoms include: Coagulopathy; hepatic encephalopathy; and esophageal varices with bleeding; spontaneous bacterial peritonitis; and refractory ascites that is not responsive to diuretics.

HEPATOCELLULAR DISEASES

Hepatocellular disease is any disease that affects the cells of the liver, including:

- **Chronic hepatitis**
  - o Hepatitis B, C and D (disallow alcohol as a co-morbid factor)
  - o Autoimmune diseases (porphyria)
  - o Iatrogenic disease from using Macrobid, Aldomet, Dopamet, and Novomedopa
- **Steatohepatitis** (fatty inflammation of the liver)
  - o Alcohol
  - o Obesity
  - o Iatrogenic disease from Cordarone
- **Vascular disease**
  - o Chronic Budd-Chiari syndrome (thrombotic or nonthrombotic obstruction of the hepatic vein)
- **Inborn errors of metabolism**
  - o Hemochromatosis (inherited disorder where the body stores too much iron)
  - o Alpha-1 Antitrypsin deficiency (genetic disorder that causes lung diseases)
  - o Wilson's disease (genetic disorder that causes the body to retain copper)
  - o Glycogen storage disease, types I and III

CHOLESTASIS

Cholestasis is a condition where the bile cannot flow from the liver to the duodenum of the small intestines. The **intrahepatic bile duct** passes through and drains bile from the liver. Diseases that affect the intrahepatic bile duct are:

- Biliary atresia (common bile duct between the liver and small intestines is blocked)
- Primary biliary cirrhosis (disease that destroys the bile ducts in the liver)
- Iatrogenic, drug-induced diseases (e.g., chlorpromazine and tolbutamide)
- Familial cholestasis (Byler's syndrome and arteriohepatic dysplasia)
- Cystic fibrosis (sticky buildup of mucus in the intestines can lead to inspissated [thickened, dried] bile syndrome and cirrhosis)

EXTRAHEPATIC BILE DUCT

The **extrahepatic bile duct** is the part of the common hepatic bile duct that joins the gallbladder though the gallbladder duct, forming the common bile duct, and carrying acids and enzymes into the small intestine to digest fatty foods. Diseases affecting these are:

- Primary sclerosing cholangitis (chronic cholestatic liver disease of unknown etiology)
- Secondary biliary cirrhosis (occurs when large bile ducts outside of the liver become blocked)
- Congenital abnormalities
- Urea cycle enzyme deficiency (deficiency in enzymes responsible for removing ammonia from the blood)
- Homozygous hypercholesterolemia (very rare disease characterized by accelerated, severe atherosclerosis)
- Primary Hyperoxaluria Type I (overproduction of oxalate, a salt that binds strongly with calcium)
- Familial amyloidotic polyneuropathy (genetic disorder where the body produces a mutation of a protein found in the liver)
- Developmental abnormalities
- Polycystic liver disease (many cysts scattered throughout the liver, causing massive hepatomegaly)
- Caroli's disease (very rare disease which causes dilation of the biliary tree)

CAUSES OF ESRD IN THE UNITED STATES

There are three **main causes of end-stage renal disease (ESRD)** in the U.S.: Diabetes, hypertension, and glomerulonephritis. At present, diabetes mellitus is the number one cause of ESRD. Recent studies indicate that development of nephropathy is linked genetic predisposition, age, hypertension, gender, high blood sugar levels, smoking, and ethnicity. Patient education on controllable factors is imperative (smoking, hypertension, and blood glucose levels). Glomerulonephritis is a degenerative condition in which the kidney's filtration system is inflamed, has scar tissue, and is no longer able to properly remove body waste efficiently. Glomerulonephritis leads to high blood pressure, which in turn leads to progressive loss of kidney function.

COMMON DISEASES THAT NECESSITATE A KIDNEY OR KIDNEY-PANCREAS TRANSPLANT

Diseases requiring kidney transplant include polycystic kidney disease, primary glomerulonephritis, HIV-associated nephropathy, glomerulonephritis, diabetic nephropathy, hypertension, systemic lupus erythematosus, other systemic diseases, and other genetic diseases.

16

Diseases requiring kidney-pancreas transplant include end-stage diabetic nephropathy, life-threatening Type I diabetes (IDDM), and life-threatening hypoglycemia.

REASONS FOR INTESTINAL TRANSPLANT

Intestinal transplants primarily involve the small intestine, rather than the colon. The colon excretes mostly water and fiber as stools, and can be efficiently replaced with a colostomy bag. Prior to considering a small bowel transplant, physicians give the patient total parenteral nutrition (TPN). Functional failure of the small intestine means either the patient is unable to properly absorb nutrients from TPN, or has severe complications related to the motility of the intestine. Intestinal complications can occur at any age from:

- **Structural diseases:** Crohn's disease; small bowel stenosis; necrotizing enterocolitis; trauma; vascular accidents; mesenteric thrombosis; atresia or stenosis of the small intestine
- **Functional complications:** Congenital enteritis; total intestinal aganglionosis; and radiation enteritis.

REASONS FOR PERFORMING INTESTINAL TRANSPLANTS IN ADULTS

The indications for intestinal transplantation vary greatly from adult to pediatric populations. In **adults**, the two leading causes for transplantation are Crohn's disease and vascular insufficiency.

- **Crohn's disease**, also known as regional enteritis, is chronic episodes of inflammation of the gastrointestinal tract, characterized by transmural inflammation and cobblestoning. Crohn's disease can involve any area of the GI tract, and ranges from mild to severe. In severe cases, TPN is needed for nutritional support after bowel resection.
- **Vascular insufficiency** results from: A hypercoagulable state; veno-occlusive disorder; familial adenomatous polyposis (develop and progression of intestinal polyps associated with a pre-cancerous state); radiation enteritis (intestinal damage due to radiation); and injury.

DISEASES IN CHILDREN

Children with Hirschsprung disease and chronic intestinal pseudo-obstruction (CIP) are most likely to need an intestinal transplant.

- **Hirschsprung disease** is also known as congenital aganglionic megacolon. There is an enlargement of the colon, in conjunction with improper peristalsis (muscle movements), which result in an intestinal obstruction. Patients present with abdominal bloating, severe constipation or recurrent fecal impaction, anemia, and malnutrition.
- **Chronic intestinal pseudo-obstruction (CIP)** also results from ineffective peristalsis, but occurs in the absence of an intestinal obstruction. CIP is usually discovered at birth or by one year of age. CIP can involve the entire intestinal tract or just a section. The most common presenting signs and symptoms are abdominal bloating, infrequent passage of hard stools, and vomiting bile.

STRUCTURAL INDICATIONS IN CHILDREN

Volvulus and gastroschisis are the two most common **structural causes** of intestinal transplantation in **children**.

- A **volvulus** occurs when a segment of the small intestine loops around itself as a result of adhesions, congenital deformity, or twisting of the mesentery, resulting in vascular insufficiency. Volvulus is most often discovered in utero or shortly after birth. However, volvulus can occur in any age group.
- **Gastroschisis** is also called laparoschisis. It occurs when an abdominal wall defect appears, usually on the right side. The intestines and other abdominal organs herniate into a small abdominal cavity, or protrude outside of the abdominal wall. Gastroschisis is seen in premature infants. Their intestines look short and swollen because they were exposed to amniotic fluid.

Less common structural indications that require children to undergo intestinal transplantation are **congenital atresia** (narrowing of the small intestine), **necrotizing enterocolitis (NEC)**, and **trauma**.

SHORT GUT SYNDROME

Intestinal transplants are usually performed on both adults and children as a result of **short gut syndrome (SGS),** the inability of the small intestines to adequately absorb nutrition, fluids, and to regulate electrolytes. SGS is usually an acquired condition. However, in rare cases, children are born this way. SGS can result in malabsorption, hypersecretory state, poor growth and development, and an inability to sustain weight. SGS is classified into two categories: Structural and functional. Structural SGS is the consequence of an extensive surgical resection of the small intestines, or an anatomic anomaly featuring a considerable reduction in the length of the small intestines. Functional SGS patients may have a satisfactory small intestinal length, but the intestine fails to properly take up nutrients, produce important GI secretions, or sustain sufficient peristalsis.

DISEASES THAT NECESSITATE A HEART TRANSPLANT

Common diseases necessitating a **heart transplant** include the following:

- Congenital heart conditions
- Congestive heart failure with:
  - Class III-IV symptoms
  - On maximum therapy
  - Reduced exercise capacity
  - Severe oxygen dependence of < 14 ml/kg/min
- End-stage heart disease
- Heart valve disease
- Myocarditis
- Myxomas (heart tumor)
- Refractory angina despite therapeutic interventions
- Restrictive, dilated, or ischemic cardiomyopathy
- Life-threatening ventricular arrhythmias

Pre-Transplant Evaluation Process

PRE-TRANSPLANT EVALUATION PROCESS

The potential recipient must undergo an extensive medical-surgical and psychosocial **evaluation prior to acceptance on the transplantation waiting list.** This evaluation uses a *multidisciplinary approach* (takes into consideration viewpoints from different disciplines; holistic). Essential components considered include: Past medical history; current illnesses; past surgical history; family history; current medications; psychosocial history; and current physical state. Key elements of the pre-transplant evaluation process include establishing the:

- Cause of end-organ disease.
- Possibility for transplantation.
- Contraindications to transplantation.
- Risk for recurrent disease in the allograft.
- Likelihood of the donor and recipient withstanding the rigors of transplant surgery.
- Comorbidities that may affect the post-transplant path or recovery process.
- Donor's and recipient's capability of withstanding immunosuppressive therapy.
- Identification of all possible living donors, unless a good volunteer match is already on offer.

DIAGNOSTIC TESTS

Diagnostic tests performed during the pre-transplant evaluation include:

- **Abdominal ultrasound:** Examine the patient for gallstones and any other abnormal findings or disease processes.
- **Chest X-ray:** Evaluate the patient's lung condition, and check for cardiomegaly (enlarged heart) or any other abnormal findings.
- **Electrocardiogram (EKG):** Evaluate the patient's heart rate and rhythm. If it is not normal sinus rhythm, then order a Holter monitor for arrhythmia evaluation.
- **Panorex:** Examine the teeth and jaws for cavities, abscesses, and gingivitis that may cause a post-transplant infection.
- **Pulmonary function test (PFT):** Measure how much air the patient's lungs can hold, how fast air can be moved in and out of the patient's lungs, and how well the lungs retain oxygen and discard carbon dioxide.
- Purified protein derivative (PPD): Test for tuberculosis (TB).
- **Right heart catheterization** (only if needed): Assess the pressure inside the patient's heart.

> **Review Video: EKG Rhythms - Reading the Graph**
> Visit mometrix.com/academy and enter code: 872282

PRE-TRANSPLANT LAB TESTS

Pre-transplant labs include the following:

- **ABO blood typing:** Per the UNOS requirements, two separate tests are conducted on two separate occasions.
- **Panel Reactive Antibody**: PRA calculates the probability of developing rejection following transplantation.
- **Human Leukocyte Antigen:** HLA predicts organ rejection.

- **Virology screening:** Includes HIV, hepatitis, herpes, CMV, and EBV. Determines suitability for transplantation and post-transfusion infection risk.
- **Toxoplasma screening:** Organ recipients risk developing reactivation toxoplasmosis post-transplantation if they: Received an organ from a toxoplasmosis-infected donor; had past exposure to protozoa-infected cat feces; ate undercooked lamb, pork, or venison; were accidentally inoculated by working in a lab; or contracted toxoplasmosis from their mothers during pregnancy.
- **Cancer screening:** Immunosuppressives like Cyclosporin, taken to reduce graft rejection, increase the cancer risk for recipients.
- **Osteoporosis screening:** Recipients risk osteoporosis and bone fractures because they take steroids, heparin, and loop diuretics.
- **Tuberculosis (TB) screening:** TB causes the potential organ recipient to become *anergic*.

PRE-TRANSPLANT VIROLOGY SCREENING

Virology screening is blood or swab tests conducted on all pre-transplant recipients to determine if they are suitable for organ transplantation, and if they have any associated post-transplant risk factors:

Disease	Initial Screening Test
HIV	Enzyme immunoassay test (ELISA)
Hepatitis A, B, and C	HBsAg, Anti-HAV IgM, HAV IgM Ab, EIA
Herpes Virus Screening	HSV-1 (Alphaherpesvirinae), HSV-2, herpes virus antigen or antibody, herpes viral culture
Cytomegalovirus	CMV (Betaherpesvirinae)
Epstein Barr virus (mononucleosis)	Monospot (heterophile antibody)

PANEL REACTIVE ANTIBODY

Panel Reactive Antibody (PRA) is a blood test commonly performed on all potential solid organ transplant patients. PRA determines the recipient's sensitivity to a donor's antigens by measuring anti-human antibodies in blood using a percentage from 0% to 99%. The higher the PRA percentage, the higher the number of antibodies found, which increases the risk of post-transplant rejection, morbidity, and mortality. For example, if a recipient's PRA is 75%, it means the antibodies in the recipient's blood would bind to the tissue types of 75% of the donors in the population. The recipient is limited to receiving a donation from the remaining 25% of the population, which decreases the likelihood of a transplant match. People who have received numerous blood transfusions are more likely to have high PRA levels.

HUMAN LEUKOCYTE ANTIGEN

Human Leukocyte Antigen (HLA) is a pre-transplant blood test that detects protein markers (antigens) on the surface of most cells, including white blood cells. Red blood cells and CNS cells do not have HLA. Protein markers are used in the discrimination process of identifying self from non-self. HLA is used pre-operatively to predict the likelihood of organ rejection. HLA located on the surface of the white blood cells plays an essential role in the body's immune system and inflammatory response. HLA is a test requirement of the United Network for Organ Sharing (UNOS) and the European transplant registries lists. The HLA test is highly sensitive to detecting antigens, so the test cannot be performed if a blood transfusion has occurred within the past 72 hours. The genes on chromosome 6 are responsible for the major histocompatibility complex (MHC), of which HLA is a part.

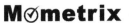

Exceptions When HIV Positive Person May Be Considered for a Solid Organ Transplant

The topic of **HIV positive persons receiving solid organ donations** is hotly debated because HIV is often the cause of chronic liver and renal disease. Due to recent medical advances, a person with HIV can now expect to live longer (~10 years after diagnosis). Some transplant centers will consider solid organ donations for HIV patients who meet the following criteria:

- CD4 cell count is greater than 200 cells per cubic millimeter of blood for longer than six months.
- Levels of HIV ribonucleic acid (RNA) are undetectable.
- HIV has not progressed to AIDS.
- Compliance (consistently taking HIV medications as prescribed by a physician for more than 3 months).
- No opportunistic infections related to HIV diagnosis.

Absolute Contraindications

Absolute contraindications are factors that always exclude a person from receiving a solid organ transplant, regardless of the state in which the organ is located or transplant center location. The most common absolute contraindications for solid organ transplantation are:

- Active drinker, smoker, or drug user.
- AIDS or HIV positive (an HIV positive diagnosis is no longer an absolute contraindication in a growing number of localities)
- Any active infection.
- Cancer (active or recent history).
- Irreversible damage to any organ other than the organ needed for transplantation.
- Diverticulitis.
- "Free Bleeder" or difficulty clotting.
- History of non-compliance.
- Mental disorders.
- Pulmonary embolism.
- Stomach Ulcers (PUD).

Absolute contraindications to transplants may vary somewhat according to the type of transplant:

- **Heart**: Severe pulmonary hypertension (irreversible), severe systemic illness, advanced obstructive pulmonary disease, active malignancy, substance abuse, and inadequate support system.
- **Kidney**: Vascular anatomy inadequacy, severe cardiopulmonary disease, BMI >40 kg/m², inadequate support system, and active malignancy, infection, or substance abuse.
- **Liver**: Severe cardiopulmonary disease, inadequate support system, active malignancy, unstable mental illness, unstable HIV, non-compliance with treatments, current substance abuse, and inadequate anatomic features.
- **Lungs**: Malignancy within 2 years, unstable systemic illness of other organs, chronic infection (HIV, hepatitis), inadequate anatomic features, unstable mental health, inadequate support system, and substance abuse (current or within 6 months, including cigarettes).

- **Pancreas/Islet cells:** Frequently done simultaneously with kidney transplant or following kidney transplant, so patients must meet those same criteria. Contraindications are similar and include malignancy (within 2 years), inadequate social support, non-compliance with treatment, aortoiliac vascular disease, severe coronary artery disease, and severe malnutrition.

PAIRED EXCHANGE, INDIRECT EXCHANGE, AND NON-DIRECTED DONATION

A **paired exchange** consists of two living donors who are agreeable to donate one kidney each, but they do not meet the ABO compatibility requirements for their chosen recipients. An uncomplicated exchange takes place, coordinated by the transplant center. The donors donate to the recipients with whom they are compatible, but they do not necessarily know each other.

An **indirect exchange** occurs when one living kidney donor is prepared to donate, but does not meet the ABO compatibility requirement. The living donor donates to the first person on the transplant waiting list for a cadaveric kidney who is ABO compatible. In exchange for this anonymous donation, the donor's originally planned recipient is moved to the top of the waiting list for a cadaveric kidney.

A **non-directed donation** transpires when a living donor offers a kidney to the transplant center as a Good Samaritan. Non-direct donors do not have anyone particular in mind that they would like to receive their donated kidney. The donation is usually anonymous.

ORGANS DONATED BY LIVING DONORS AND ENDURING HEALTH EFFECTS

The following **organs can be donated by a living donor**: Kidneys; liver lobes; lung lobes; pancreas segments; and small bowel segments. Note that small bowel segment donations have had limited success to-date. The combined research on kidney donors spans more than 30 years, and kidney transplant technology is quite advanced, so kidney donors experience few or no enduring effects on their physical health. However, there is some data to support the development of depression in kidney donors. The depression stems from feelings of being forgotten, unwanted or insignificant, or a sense of being exploited. Liver and lung transplants are much newer than kidney transplants. There is not as much long-term follow-up research to use as a reference. However, there have not been any long-term effects of significant concern reported in the literature.

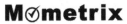

Patient Monitoring While Awaiting Transplant

NEXT STEP AFTER PRE-TRANSPLANT EVALUATION

Each patient is individually considered for organ donation because of the complexity of interacting risk factors. Once all lab tests have been completed for the potential recipient and the written results are available, the multidisciplinary team meets to discuss all findings in a group setting. Each member makes arrangements for special needs, in anticipation of an organ becoming available. Once the multidisciplinary team reaches a decision, they notify the patient, family, and attending physician. The patient may be:

- Accepted as an organ recipient and placed on a cadaveric (dead donor) waiting list.
- Scheduled for immediate surgery if an organ is available from a live donor.
- Denied based on qualifying criteria.
- Temporarily deferred due to discrepancies found during the evaluation process.

ELEMENTS MONITORED IN PATIENT AWAITING TRANSPLANT

Elements that must be monitored in a patient **awaiting transplant** include:

- Changes in health status that may affect outcomes.
- Changes in health insurance or support system that may preclude transplantation.
- Changes in contact information (address, telephone number, texting number).
- Availability and ability to go to transplant center immediately or within several hours if an organ becomes available for transplant.
- Laboratory testing (organ-specific) to ensure the patient remains eligible for transplant. May include walk tests, echocardiogram, cardiac stress test, chest x-ray, blood tests, ABGs, panel reactive antibody.
- Immunizations: Must be current to reduce the risk of infection.
- Substance abuse: Includes alcohol and drugs and (in some cases) smoking. Those with relapses may be removed from wait list temporarily or permanently.
- Emotional/Mental status of patient and support providers.
- Exercise programs or rehabilitation programs to maintain the patient in optimal condition.

KARNOFSKY PERFORMANCE STATUS

The **Karnofsky Performance Status Scale** (KPS) classifies clients according to their functional abilities and impairments with scores ranging from 100 (normal with no indications of disease) to 0 (death). The KPS score of patients receiving transplants must be reported to UNOS. KPS scale is used to determine risk-adjusted outcomes and survival rates for transplant centers.

Condition	Score	Functional ability
Independent in care	100	No evidence of disease or health complaints
	90	Able to carry out ADLs but has minor symptoms.
	80	Able to carry out ADLs with effort, some signs/symptoms.
Inability to work but ability to live at home with some assistance	70	Can manage self-care, but cannot carry out normal activities or do active work.
	60	Needs occasional help with self-care.
	50	Needs much assistance and frequent medical care.
Need for institutionalization or hospitalization	40	Disabled and needs special care and assistance.
	30	Disabilities severe, needs hospitalization but not terminal.
	20	Severely ill, requires hospitalization and active support.
	10	Dying.
	0	Deceased.

Things Patients Awaiting Transplant Must Avoid

Patients **awaiting transplantation** must avoid:

- Engaging in substance abuse (may include smoking). Patients generally must be free of substance abuse for specified periods (6 months to 2 years) and may be removed from wait list temporarily or permanently if relapses occur.
- Non-compliance with treatment regimen, including not only medications but also diet and exercise programs.
- Failing to keep medical appointments or completing medical testing as required. This may be complicated if the patient is registered with more than one transplant center, and some centers may require retesting.
- Inadequate preparation: The patient must be educated about the transplant and requirements of the wait list and should make a financial plan for living arrangements and transportation if the transplant center is located at a distance.
- Losing hope: The patient needs to hold onto hope and motivation in order to survive until a transplant becomes available.

Priorities for Patients Awaiting Transplants

Priorities for patients awaiting transplant include:

- Carrying cell phone at all times in case an organ becomes available.
- Adhering to all treatment regimens and keeping all medical appointments.
- Maintaining emotional/mental health, by using open communication with family/friends, attending support groups when available, and finding methods to manage stress.

- Maintaining readiness: Keeping updated transportation plans and housing plans, having bags packed and ready to go, and ensuring a 24-hour supply of medications and IV solution (if necessary) is always readily available.
- Carrying a medication list with all current medications and dosages listed as well as contact numbers for physicians and other healthcare providers.
- Preparing advance directives and informing family members of wishes regarding end-of-life care and DNR.
- Maintaining insurance and notifying the transplant center of any changes.
- Avoiding substance abuse of any kind.
- Avoiding exposure to infectious diseases and keeping immunizations current.
- Obtaining financial assistance if needed.

WAITING LIST PROCESS FOR ORGAN TRANSPLANTATION

The national transplant **waiting list** is managed by the United Network for Organ Sharing (UNOS). Before being placed on the waiting list, a patient must be evaluated by a transplant center to ensure the patient meets the criteria and has the supports (emotional, physical, financial) necessary. Once accepted as a candidate for transplantation, information (blood and tissue type, medical urgency, distance to transplant center, and body size) about a candidate is entered into the UNOS database to facilitate matching when an organ comes available. When an organ is procured from an Organ Procurement Organization (OPO), UNOS is notified and the matching process begins to determine who on the waiting list is a match for the organ. Out of that pool, the most appropriate candidate is selected. Classifications systems may vary depending on the organ needed. For example, the UNOS classification for those needing a heart includes:

- 1A: Urgent need, in intensive care and requires life-saving treatment.
- IB: Needs IV medications and/or mechanical-assist device. May be hospitalized or maintained at home.
- 2: On oral medications and stable, not hospitalized.
- 7/Inactive: Not currently in need of transplant.

Preparing the Pre-Transplant Patient

PRE-TRANSPLANT PSYCHOSOCIAL EVALUATION

Psychosocial evaluation areas that must be looked at closely include:

- **Compliance:** Does the patient have a history of non-compliance with medication and/or a health regimen? Ask about compliance with diet, exercise, fluid restrictions, keeping doctors' appointments, etc.
- **Substance abuse:** Inquire about past and present use of tobacco products, alcohol consumption, and recreational drug use. Ask about any prior rehab stays, AAA meetings, etc.
- **Mental Status:** Is the patient alert and oriented X 3 (to time, place, and person)? Look for any unusual cognitive behaviors, such as difficulty remembering the past, or showing a lack of concentration.
- **Support Factors:** Inquire about family dynamics, the patient's support structure, and its stability, e.g., friends, housing, finances, religious affiliation, etc.
- **Health Perspective:** How does the patient view his or her medical condition? What are the patient's personal expectations? What expectations does the patient's family have? Do they realize immunosuppressives will be necessary long term, and that they can cause serious complications? Are the expectations unrealistic?

The following are specific **psychosocial components** evaluated in the potential recipient:

- **Demographics:** Patient's age, number of children and their ages, and patient's marital status.
- **Support structure:** Number of people in the patient's direct support structure and specific supports each person provides.
- **Emotional status:** Any history of mental illness, especially depression and suicide attempts.
- **Health behaviors:** Patient's history of follow-up with routine doctor appointments, and current medical requirements such as oxygen canisters or dialysis machine.
- **Home environment:** Assess the home environment's overall condition, and look for the presence of stairs, a telephone, plumbing, electricity, a furnace, and an air conditioner. Does the patient own or rent? Is the home an apartment, house, or mobile home?
- **Social habits:** History and current use of alcohol, tobacco, and drugs.
- **Coping skills:** How well the patient deals with difficult situations.
- **Cognitive level:** Comprehension level and ability to understand information presented, including reading and educational levels.
- **Transportation:** Ability to travel to all medical appointments (both scheduled and un-scheduled).
- **Finances:** The patient's health insurance coverage, savings account, and source of income.

SOCIAL AND PSYCHOPATHOLOGICAL FACTORS THAT MAY CONTRIBUTE TO DENIAL OF TRANSPLANTATION

The **rate of denial** varies greatly and takes into account multiple factors, judged on an individual basis, which may ultimately have no bearing on the final decision. If the patient has any of the following, he/she is unlikely to be transplanted:

- Is not currently a citizen of the United States.
- Is not a state resident where the transplant facility is located.
- Is currently serving a prison sentence or has an extensive criminal history.
- Recently lost a loved one.

- Recently endured a great loss, like bankruptcy or destruction of a home.
- Has an active or controlled mental health condition, such as Alzheimer's disease, dementia, schizophrenia, bipolar disorder, severe depression, history of suicide attempts, intellectual disability, etc.

CROSSMATCHING

Crossmatching is usually the final test conducted just prior to the transplant. Crossmatching identifies reactivity between the serum of the organ recipient and lymphocytes from the organ donor. A positive crossmatch signifies that the organ recipient has HLA antibody directed against the donor's tissue, which could cause early graft rejection. Crossmatching is performed prior to transplantation on all renal recipients, and post-transplantation for all liver recipients. Heart, lung, and pancreas transplant recipients usually are crossmatched after transplantation, unless the PRA is greater than 10%-15%. In that instance, the crossmatch may be performed prior to transplantation.

MATCHING ANTIGEN SYSTEMS

An organ recipient and organ donor must have two antigen systems matched: Blood group and type (**ABO Rh**), and **HLA**. If a recipient receives the wrong organ or blood match, **ABO Rh reaction** causes hyperacute rejection with rigors (severe chills and fever), back and joint pain, difficulty breathing, stomach upset, oozing wounds, apprehension, and shock from circulatory collapse (hypotension). Patients with a **hemolytic reaction** from an incompatible blood group develop disseminated intravascular coagulation (**DIC**), renal failure, and death. **Human leukocyte alloimmunization reaction** causes organ rejection because the recipient's HLA system destroys the foreign donor transplant. Generally, irradiated blood does not need to be given to solid organ transplant patients. However, irradiated blood products prevent fatal transfusion-associated graft-versus-host disease (**TAGVHD**) in: Bone marrow recipients; donors who require autologous transfusion; direct donors; HLA-matched platelet recipients; family members who are donor and recipient; fetuses and premature babies; and cancer patients with glioblastoma; Hodgkin's disease; leukemia; lymphoma; neuroblastoma; and T-cell deficiency.

PATIENT PREPARATION FOR TRANSPLANTATION SURGERY

Patient preparation for transplantation surgery, beginning at the time of notification, includes:

- Initiating procedures as outlined in transplantation plan, including notifying significant others, transporting to the transplantation center, and bringing all necessary medications, medication lists, equipment, personal care items (toothbrush, denture containers, deodorants, hearing aids), ID cards, and insurance cards.
- Bringing advance directives to the transplantation center and ensuring that family members are aware of wishes.
- Following all preoperative directions regarding food and fluid restrictions and medications.
- Contacting spiritual/religious supports, such as priests, ministers, imams, rabbis, if desired so they can provide emotional support.
- Asking questions as needed to ensure complete understanding of rights, responsibilities, procedures, risks and benefits, and to ensure the ability to give informed consent.
- Cooperating with all testing and assessments required preoperatively.
- Reporting immediately any recent changes in condition or signs of infection or complications.

- Beginning antirejection medications if prescribed.
- Bathing, showering with special soap if so indicated (usually the evening before and morning of surgery).

PATIENT PREPARATION THE DAY OF SURGERY

Patient preparation on the day of surgery will vary depending on the patient's condition, on whether the patient is already hospitalized, and on the type of transplantation that will be carried out. Some common preparations for the patient include:

- Removing jewelry and showering with special antiseptic soap.
- Taking oral medications that are allowed with a sip of water.
- Arriving at the transplant center at least 2 hours before scheduled surgery.

Common **preparations for nursing and medical staff** include:

- Reassuring the patient and providing information.
- Verifying NPO status and medications.
- Advising family where they can wait and how they will receive information.
- Final crossmatching to ensure that the organ matches the recipient.
- Taking the patient to the preoperative area.
- Carrying out any prep, such as shaving, that is required.
- Starting an IV line and administering any medications (such as sedatives) as directed.
- Transporting patient to the operating room.

RECOMMENDED IMMUNIZATIONS PRIOR TO ORGAN TRANSPLANTATION

Any infection that occurs after a solid organ transplant is of great concern, due to the patient's depressed immune state. Post-transplant infection is a significant cause of grave illness and death (morbidity and mortality). The best way to prevent pre-and-post-transplant infections is by **immunizations** for:

- Flu (influenza)
- Hepatitis A (liver recipients)
- Hepatitis B (all organ recipients)
- Pneumonia (Pneumococcus)

All *live* vaccines must be administered several months prior to organ transplantation, and must be given to both the recipient *and* family members living in the same home as the organ recipient. Three examples of live vaccines are MMR, varicella-zoster, and oral polio.

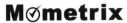

Post-Transplant Care

POST-OPERATIVE ASSESSMENT FOR NEUROCOGNITIVE DEFICITS

Not all transplant recipients will experience **post-transplant cognitive impairment**. However, unless the recipient complains about being unable to think clearly, post-transplant neurocognitive deficits may go unnoticed. Patients may "fake good" at follow-up visits, but have difficulty coping at home due to mental cloudiness or confusion. If a recipient exhibits signs of noncompliance with therapy or the recovery regimen, assess his or her comprehension level on these topics. With the recipient's consent, ask family members if they notice any cognitive behavioral changes post-transplant. If cognitive deficits are present, refer the recipient immediately to a specialist for neurocognitive testing. Educate the recipient and family about strategies to help minimize any neurological effects.

IMMUNE TOLERANCE AND COSTIMULATION

Immune tolerance is when the body accepts a foreign object as "self" and does not launch an immune response against it. For an organ transplant to be successful, the body must accept the donor organ as non-foreign.

Costimulation is a new and very appealing approach to immunosuppression because *it does not suppress the body's entire immune system, so the body is still able to fight off bacterial and viral infections normally.* Costimulation targets only the immune response associated with the donor organ. Costimulation is a complicated process by which the communication between the T-helper cells and the APC's (antigen presenting cells) are disrupted. This disruption causes an incomplete activation of the immune system. Costimulation may be the method of choice to prevent organ rejection in the future.

TRANSPLANT ORGAN REJECTION

Transplant organ rejection is a complex process that occurs when the body's immune system detects the newly transplanted organ as non-self and attacks it. When the immune system labels something as foreign, it launches a series of attacks against it using white blood cells and antibodies. The white blood cells and antibodies are unable to attack the organ as a whole. Instead, they attack individual cells that comprise the organ tissue. This sophisticated attack causes tissue death (necrosis) of the newly transplanted organ. Using proper HLA (human leukocyte antigen) matching can help avoid transplant rejection.

HYPERACUTE REJECTION AND EARLY ACCELERATED REJECTION

Hyperacute rejection is the most devastating form of organ rejection. Hyperacute rejection is an immune-mediated response in which the recipient either has pre-existing antibodies to the donor organ, or has been ABO mismatched. Hyperacute rejection usually occurs within minutes of the transplant, but may not be noticed for hours. Once this type of rejection is identified, the donor organ must be removed immediately. This type of rejection is especially risky with kidney transplants.

Early accelerated rejection is the next concern if hyperacute rejection is not present. Early accelerated rejection occurs from 24 hours post-transplant to several days afterwards, and usually is a result of *anamnestic rejection* (rapid antibody response on the second exposure). Anamnestic rejection primarily happens when a fetus has an HLA exposure from the mother, and sensitization develops in utero. When the baby later receives an organ transplant, it is rejected. Older recipients who have had previous blood transfusions or a previous organ transplant are also likely to develop early accelerated rejection.

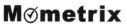

ACUTE AND CHRONIC REJECTION

Acute organ rejection occurs from days to months after an organ transplant as a result of the body's T-cells responding to detected foreign proteins from the donor organ (histocompatibility). Acute organ rejection can be greatly decreased by taking **immunosuppressive medications**, like Cyclosporin, prednisone, Imuran, Prograf, CellCept, Rapamune, ATGAM & Thymoglobulin. A single episode of acute organ rejection is not of great concern if prompt treatment is given. About 60% of kidney and liver recipients develop acute organ rejection. However, if left untreated, organ failure can result.

Chronic rejection is more subtle than acute or hyperacute rejection, so it is more difficult to diagnose and treat. Chronic rejection occurs slowly, over the course of one or more years post-transplant. **Once chronic rejection occurs, immunosuppressive therapy is usually of no help.** The effects will eventually result in total organ loss.

DIAGNOSIS OF ACUTE REJECTION IN A SOLID ORGAN TRANSPLANT

Acute rejection diagnoses vary with the different organs. Diagnosis is not typically made using one test, but rather a series of diagnostic methods. Routine surveillance tests should be conducted to diagnose rejection before a patient even becomes symptomatic. At present, tissue biopsy remains the definitive diagnostic tool for both routine surveillance and suspected rejection. The severity of acute rejection determines if treatment is necessary. Each organ has descriptive criteria that determines the severity of rejection. Adjunctive diagnostic tests are used for organ-specific diagnosis. Examples are as follows:

- Heart: Perform an echocardiogram to determine cardiac function.
- Liver: Compare present liver function tests to baseline results.

CAUSES OF POST-TRANSPLANT OCCULT FEVER

Occult fever occurs when a patient has an elevated temperature, but the cause of that elevation is unknown. The most common causes of post-transplant fever are broken down into three time periods:

- **Month 1:** Fever is usually the cause of a complication related to the surgery itself, such as infection from an indwelling bladder catheter tube. A second common cause of fever during the first month is allograft rejection (HLA histocompatibility). **Antilymphocyte therapy** with OKT3 and antilymphocyte globulin is a potential cause of occult fever, especially during the first few and last doses of a 10-14 day course. Conventional drug fevers are uncommon.
- **Months 2-6:** Antilymphocyte therapy and viral infections are common causes of occult fever during this time frame, especially Cytomegalovirus (CMV), post-transplant lymphoproliferative disorder (PTLD), and Kaposi's sarcoma.
- **More than 6 months:** Antilymphocyte therapy and **opportunistic infections**, like pneumococcal pneumonia, urinary tract infections (UTI), varicella zoster, and influenza, cause the patient's temperature to spike.

Specific Organ Transplantation Care

Lung Transplant

LUNG TRANSPLANT MEDICAL EVALUATION

Medical tests usually ordered for a potential lung transplant candidate include:

- Chest x-ray PA and lateral.
- Quantitative ventilation-perfusion scan (VQ scan) divided into two sections: The patient is *injected* with a small amount of contrast medium IV. As the contrast moves into the arteries of the lungs, the level of illumination indicates which lung receives a greater blood supply. The patient *inhales* contrast medium to indicate which lung takes in more oxygen during inspiration. Looking at both parts of the VQ scan provides important information on which lung is more affected by the disease process. The transplant team then decides on a single-lung or double-lung transplant.
- 12 lead electrocardiogram (EKG).
- Transesophageal echocardiogram (Sound waves are emitted by a small electrode inserted into the patient's esophagus. The echogram analyzes the structures of the heart and surrounding vessels.)
- Pulmonary function tests (PFT).
- Arterial blood gases (ABG).
- Oxygen desaturation study.
- Six-minute walking distance.
- Dual-energy x-ray absorptiometry (DEXA) scan.

CRITERIA FOR SINGLE-LUNG OR DOUBLE-LUNG TRANSPLANT

Objective and subjective factors are used to decide when the time is right for a lung transplant. The patient must meet these criteria:

- Life expectancy is less than 24-36 months without a transplant (objective).
- Lung disease can potentially affect the patient's other organs (objective).
- Quality of life has deteriorated significantly because of diseased lungs (subjective)

When taking these factors into account, the risk versus benefits must be carefully weighed.

Single-lung transplant	Double-lung transplant
COPD or emphysema (45%)	Cystic fibrosis (33%)
Idiopathic pulmonary fibrosis (22%)	Other causes
Alpha Antitrypsin Deficiency (11%)	Alpha Antitrypsin Deficiency
Primary pulmonary hypertension (5%)	Primary pulmonary hypertension
Other causes (17%)	Easier to transplant *both* lungs and heart from a cadaver to preserve the vessels

PHYSIOLOGICAL FACTORS THAT LIMIT CHANCES FOR RECEIVING TRANSPLANT

If a patient has these **physiological factors**, he or she is unlikely to receive a lung transplant:

- Age over 45 for heart-lung, or over 55 for bilateral lungs, or over 65 for a single lung.
- Coronary artery disease involving more than one vessel.

- Active collagen vascular disease (lupus, scleroderma, dermatomyositis, polyarteritis, rheumatoid arthritis).
- Creatinine clearance less than 50 ml/min.
- Dependent on 20 mg or more corticosteroid each day.
- Uncontrolled, brittle diabetes.
- Ejection fraction less than 20%.
- Hepatitis B or C.
- Upper respiratory infection.
- Ventilator-dependent and clinically unstable.

The list is not all-inclusive and does not imply a guarantee of organ rejection. However, these factors usually play a significant role in organ rejection, regardless of where the transplant center is located.

ACUTE AND CHRONIC REJECTION

Acute rejection takes place at least once in *all* lung transplant recipients, usually within the first 3 months after transplantation. Symptoms of acute lung rejection are: Coughing; shortness of breath; weakness; elevated temperature; low blood oxygen levels; pulmonary infiltrates; and pulmonary effusions. Treatment is high-dose corticosteroids and proper immunosuppressive therapy. If left untreated, chronic rejection will follow.

Chronic rejection is typically observed one year after transplantation. Chronic lung rejection causes the bronchioles to become swollen and fibrose. Inflammation can lead to complete bronchiole obstruction. Treatment is highly individualized and takes into account the recipient's current immunosuppressive regimen. Chronic lung rejection has a death rate of 40% or higher at three years post diagnosis.

Most experts agree that the best way to diagnose either acute or chronic lung rejection is through direct microscopic examination of tissue from lavage, brush, fine needle aspiration, transbronchial biopsy, or wedge biopsy. Less effective methods include chest X-ray, pulmonary function tests, and bronchoscopic examination.

INFECTIONS

Morbidity and mortality in lung transplant patients commonly result from infection in the first 3 months after transplantation. Common infections include:

Infection	Cause
Early bacterial pneumonia	Gram-negative pathogenic bacteria in the donor's lungs, usually *Pseudomonas, Enterobacter, Staphylococcus, Enterococcus, Hemophilus*
Late bacterial pneumonia	Develops 3 months-3 years post-transplant, usually from *Pneumococcus, Staphylococcus aureus,* and Gram-negative rods
Clostridium difficile	Excessive use of antibiotics and steroids
Fungal	*Aspergillus, Candida, Cryptococcus, Coccidioides,* or *Pseudallescheria* in the anastomosis
Viral	Usually *Cytomegalovirus, Herpes simplex, Adenovirus,* or *Epstein-Barr virus*
Parasites	Usually *Pneumocystis carinii* pneumonia (PCP), also called *Pneumocystis jiroveci.*

If a lung recipient develops a post-operative infection, 80% of the time it occurs in the donor lung, mediastinum, or pleural space. Lung transplant recipients are **high risk** because of:

- Nosocomial infections on hospital premises.
- Loss of nerve supply (denervation) during surgery results in a decreased cough reflex.
- Disruption of lymphatic drainage.
- Latent donor infections are reactivated in the immunosuppressed recipient.
- Prolonged intubation time.
- Bacterial colonization of the anastomosis.
- Airway dehiscence.
- Post-obstructive infections.
- Bronchial stenosis.
- Mediastinitis.
- Native lung occult infections.

BACTERIAL INFECTIONS SPECIFIC TO LUNG ALLOGRAFTS POST-TRANSPLANTATION

Bacteria are the primary cause of infection in post-transplant recipients. Pneumonia accounts for 60% of bacterial infections in all lung transplant recipients. The most common **bacterial pathogens** are:

- Gram-negative bacteria
  - Enterobacteriaceae
  - Pseudomonas aeruginosa
- Other primary bacterial infections
  - Streptococcus pneumoniae
  - Haemophilus influenzae
  - Staphylococcus aureus

The allograft lung is prone to infection because of an impaired cough reflex, inflammation of the airway due to rejection, inadequate mucociliary clearance, ischemia, reperfusion history, and abnormal lymph drainage. In a single-lung transplant, it is possible for infection to spread from the native lung to the newly transplanted lung.

VIRAL INFECTIONS

The most troublesome of the **viral infections** for post-lung transplant recipients is cytomegalovirus (CMV), because it leads to pneumonitis with alveolar damage, inclusions, infiltrates, and bronchiolitis obliterans. Other viral infections include herpes simplex and Epstein-Barr virus (EBV). At present, there are two main ways to treat these viral infections:

- Treat everyone with prophylactic antivirals (e.g., Acyclovir, Valacyclovir and IV Ganciclovir)
- Following the discovery of antigens circulating in the blood (antigenemia), give weekly viral checks for the first 3 months post-transplantation. After 3 months, conduct monthly tests.

Heart Transplant

ORTHOTOPIC AND HETEROTOPIC HEART TRANSPLANTATION

The two **types of heart transplant** procedures are orthotopic transplantation and heterotopic transplantation.

- **Orthotopic transplantation** is the more common of the two procedures, in which the entire diseased heart is removed and replaced by a donor's heart in the normal anatomical position.
- **Heterotopic transplantation** is rarely performed because it involves great risk. The recipient's diseased heart is left in place and the donor's heart is transplanted inside the recipient's right chest cavity, commonly called *piggybacking*. The vascular structures of the recipient's and donor's hearts are connected using *end-to-side anastomosis*. End-to-side anastomosis involves connecting the aortae, superior vena cava, and pulmonary arteries. Due to the high risk of thromboembolism, heterotopic transplantation is the last resort when a normal donor heart alone could not maintain adequate right ventricular function. Examples of this are when the donor's heart is too small for the recipient, or the recipient has irreversibly elevated pulmonary pressure.

CRITERIA FOR SUITABLE HEART FOR DONATION

Here are the **primary criteria** used to determine if a heart is suitable for donation:

- Age of the donor must be less than 50 years old.
- Arterial oxygen saturation must be greater than 80% with the use of a ventilator.

Providing these two criteria are met, then these seven **secondary criteria** are assessed next. The prospective donor has:

- No current infections with the potential to become systemic.
- No cancer located outside of the cranium.
- No ventricular arrhythmias of significant concern.
- No HIV/AIDS, Hepatitis B or C.
- No history of heart disease, including a heart attack (myocardial infarction, MI) or coronary artery disease (CAD).
- No heart structural abnormalities (vegetations on the valves or ventricular hypertrophy).
- No IV drug use history.

Note: Some transplant centers will consider transplanting the heart of an older donor to an older recipient.

PHYSIOLOGICAL CONTRAINDICATIONS

At present, there are no unanimously agreed-upon contraindications for heart transplantation. Each individual organ center has its own contraindication policy. However, some **physiologic contraindications** common to most centers are:

- Active peptic ulcer disease
- Advanced age (older than 60 or 65)
- AIDS
- Any active infection
- Any co-existing disease likely to limit life expectancy

34

- Cancer of recent history or at present
- Cerebrovascular disease (stroke, TIA)
- Chronic bronchitis
- Severe COPD
- Diverticulitis of recent history or at present
- Irreversible liver disease
- Irreversible pulmonary hypertension
- Irreversible pulmonary parenchymal disease
- Irreversible kidney disease
- Myocardial inflammatory disease
- Severe muscle wasting (cachexia)
- Severe osteoporosis
- Severe obesity
- Severe peripheral vascular disease
- Systemic granulomatous disease

ROUTINE OUTPATIENT CARE WHILE ON WAITING LIST

Routine care of a **potential heart recipient** includes:

- Echocardiograms to assess the heart's current ejection fraction (EF).
- Metabolic exercise tests to see if there is still a need for a heart transplant, because on rare occasions, the heart's left ventricular function recovers without intervention.
- Monitor any significant changes in weight that may have a positive or negative impact on a heart candidate's qualifications for transplant.
- If a blood transfusion is necessary:
  - Ensure leukocyte-depleted blood is always used, or ask Blood Bank to use a leukocyte-removing filter.
  - If the recipient is cytomegalovirus-seronegative, ensure only cytomegalovirus-negative blood is used, and check the reactive antibody levels after the transfusion.
- Update immunizations per protocol.
- Monitor blood electrolytes, renal function, and liver function.

INTERVALS RECOMMENDED FOR ENDOMYOCARDIAL BIOPSIES AFTER TRANSPLANT

The guidelines for **post-transplant endomyocardial biopsies** vary. However, as a general rule, biopsies are performed more often during the first 6-12 months after a heart transplant. If the patient remains asymptomatic for a long period of time, the biopsies may be discontinued, unless complications arise. *Providing all biopsy results are normal*, a typical schedule will probably resemble the following:

Post-transplant interval	Frequency
Weeks 1-6	Weekly
Weeks 7-16	2-week intervals
Months 5-6	4-week intervals
Months 7-12	6-week intervals
Months 12-24	3-month intervals
Months 25-60	6-month intervals
After 60 months	PRN with symptoms

35

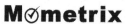

Each institution may follow a different protocol. Check the institution policies and procedures manual.

REJECTION

Rejection of a transplant heart is due to the recipient's immune system attacking and attempting to destroy the donor heart because it is foreign. The Bethesda Conference Task Force is an organization of expert physicians who set guidelines for the practice of cardiovascular medicine. BCTF defines heart rejection as "any clinical event, usually, but not always, accompanied by abnormal endomyocardial biopsy findings that is treated with significant augmentation of immunosuppression."

Type	Occurrence	Characteristics
Hyperacute	Rare; occurs immediately, in the first minutes post-transplantation	Humoral rejection; hasty tissue death is seen because of allograft failure; usually lethal
Acute	Usually occurs during first few months post-transplant	Rejection at cellular level
Chronic	More than six months post-transplant	Interstitial; insidious

ALLOGRAFT REJECTION GRADING

Grade	Histology
0	No inflammation or myocyte damage found; no rejection
1A	Perivascular or interstitial infiltrate seen, but no necrosis
1B	Sparse infiltrates found, but no necrosis
2	One focus that may be associated with myocyte damage
3A	Multifocal; may be associated with myocyte damage
3B	Diffuse mononuclear inflammation; necrosis found
4	Diffuse, aggressive polymorphous infiltrate; necrosis found; patient may have edema, bleeding, or vasculitis

IDENTIFICATION

The most recognized way of **detecting a heart transplant rejection** is through the use of a **bioptome**. A bioptome is a small catheter with a gripping device attached to one end of it. The cardiologist or surgeon uses the gripping device to remove a small piece of endomyocardial tissue for biopsy. This is a fairly simple procedure. The optimal approach involves the doctor inserting the bioptome into the right internal jugular vein. From there, the doctor advances the catheter into the right atrium, across the tricuspid valve, and into the right ventricle. If the patient's right internal jugular vein is not suitable, a second approach is to use a femoral artery.

SIGNS AND SYMPTOMS OF EARLY HEART REJECTION

Early heart rejection manifests with vague **signs and symptoms**, such as: Fatigue; shortness of breath; low-grade fever; and mood changes. Once the clinical manifestations below also present, the allograft rejection has usually advanced to a severe state.

- Cardiac arrhythmias.
- Decrease in electrocardiogram voltage.

36

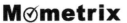

- Echocardiogram changes (decrease in systolic function, obvious modifications in the left ventricle wall or thickening of the ventricle wall, diminished left ventricular chamber size, decreased isovolemic relaxation time, enhanced early transmittal filling velocity.
- Enlarged cardiac silhouette.
- Exercise intolerance.
- Jugular vein distention.
- Lung crackles.
- New hypotension.
- New onset peripheral edema.
- Pericardial friction (commonly called a rub).
- S3 or S4 new in nature.
- Weight increase.

QUILTY EFFECT

Quilty effect (QE) is a tissue lesion found on the endocardium of a heart allograft due to lymphocytic infiltration, which has no proven clinical significance but a *strong association with acute rejection (AR) is suspected*. Quilty effect is caused primarily from the use of cyclosporin. According to the ISHLT (The International Society for Heart and Lung Transplantation), there are two patterns of Quilty lesions:

- Quilty A: Non-invasive infiltration has no effect on the underlying myocardium
- Quilty B: Invasive infiltration involves the underlying myocardium and is associated with myocyte damage

However, neither of these two types of Quilty lesions is associated with a higher incident of severe allograft rejection or survival, or coronary artery vasculopathy.

COMPLICATIONS

Complications post-transplant:

Complications	Pharmacological treatment options
High blood pressure	Calcium channel blockers; ACE inhibitors; βeta-blockers
Elevated lipid levels	Bile binding medications (Questran and Colestid); niacin; folic acid; Hydroxy-methyl-glutaryl coenzyme reductase inhibitor
Osteoporosis	Calcium; Vitamin D; substitute HCTZ for loop diuretics; and decrease steroid therapy
Diabetes	Sulfonylureas; oral hypoglycemic agents; and insulin therapy.
Kidney failure	Use *with extreme caution* any medication that increases calcineurin inhibitor levels or brings about synergistic nephrotoxicity.
GI complications	Antisecretory compounds; H2 Blockers (Tagamet; Pepcid); and replace Imuran with CellCept

POST-TRANSPLANT INFECTION

Remember these important facts regarding **infection** in post-transplant heart recipients:

- Lungs are the most common site of infection.
- All viruses are worrisome (Cytomegalovirus, Epstein-Barr virus, Herpes simplex 1 and 2, and Varicella zoster).
- Cytomegalovirus (Human Herpes Virus 5, HHV-5) is the most common cause of viral infection.
- TORCHES syndrome (toxoplasmosis, other agents, rubella, cytomegalovirus, herpes simplex, Epstein-Barr, and syphilis) is common in newborns that are small, feed poorly, are jaundiced, have petechiae and hepatosplenomegaly.
- The gastrointestinal tract is the most frequent place to become infected with cytomegalovirus.
- Cytomegalovirus pneumonia has the greatest death rate.
- Look out for bacterial pathogens, like Listeria monocytogenes, Nocardia asteroides, and Mycobacteria.

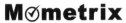

Kidney Transplant

ELIGIBILITY CRITERIA

Not everyone who has end-stage renal disease is an appropriate kidney transplant recipient. The risks and benefits of transplantation must be carefully weighed against the risks and benefits of dialysis. The decision to transplant must be motivated by medical need and patient preference. Unlike other types of organ transplants, a kidney transplant is often delayed while the patient is sustained on dialysis. A kidney transplant may be considered in certain end-stage renal patients who have a pre-dialysis creatinine clearance of less than 20 ml/min.

PHYSIOLOGICAL FACTORS THAT LIMIT CHANCES OF RECEIVING TRANSPLANT

If a patient has these **physiological factors**, he or she is unlikely to receive a **kidney** transplant:

- Benefits outweigh risks for immunosuppressive therapy versus dialysis.
- Cardiopulmonary disease.
- Hepatitis C positive, with confirmation of liver cirrhosis.
- Severe peripheral vascular disease.
- Severe abnormalities of the urinary tract system.

If a patient has these **physiological factors**, he or she is unlikely to receive a **kidney-pancreas** transplant:

- Cardiovascular disease uncorrected by surgery.
- Diabetes mellitus accompanied with severe end-stage organ damage.
- Severe peripheral vascular disease.

The lists are not all-inclusive and do not imply a guarantee of organ rejection. However, these factors usually play a significant role in organ rejection, regardless of where the transplant center is located.

LIVING RENAL DONOR

A **living renal donor** is any person who donates a kidney to someone in need of a renal transplant. The person interested in becoming a donor must take the initiative to contact a transplant center. A transplant coordinator or nurse educator will describe to the potential donor the advantages and disadvantages of donation. The potential donor must specify if the kidney is for someone in particular, or for the first match on the waiting list. The potential living renal donor must meet certain prerequisites before screening tests begin. For example, the donor must be between the ages of 18 and 65, must be healthy, have no addictions, and must be able to understand the implications of his or her decision. *If the donor decides to withdraw the offer at any time during the evaluation process, that decision must be respected and upheld.* No coercion or duress by the recipient, his or her family, or staff is permitted.

AREAS OF FOCUS IN DONOR'S MEDICAL WORK-UP PHASE

The **medical work-up phase** is a broad, wide-ranging set of exams to rule out any health issues in the donor. *If any area of concern is found, a consulting physician must give the donor clearance prior to surgery.*

- **Patient's History**
  - Cancer
  - Chronic obstructive pulmonary disease (COPD)

- o Diabetes
- o Drug/Alcohol abuse
- o Heart disease
- o Medication use
- o Systemic disease with connotation of renal involvement

- **Family History**
  - o Diabetes
  - o Hypertension
  - o Kidney disease

- **Physical Assessment**
  - o Height & weight
  - o with Body Mass Index calculation
  - o Review of body systems
  - o Cancer
  - o Infections
  - o Organ dysfunctions

BECOMING A RENAL DONOR

The **three phases of the renal pre-donation process** are: Screening, evaluation, and medical work-up.

1. The **screening** process usually takes place over the phone. Phone screening rules out high-risk donors with medical conditions such as diabetes, polycystic kidney disease, or high blood pressure.
2. The **evaluation** process begins with routine blood tests, like ABO and Rh, so that not too much time is invested in a potential donor who is not a match for the recipient.
3. If the match is compatible, then the potential donor has a full **medical work-up**. During the work-up, kidney function is determined, the overall health status of the potential donor is assessed, and renal disease-related risk factors are investigated. The potential donor then is scrutinized thoroughly by the surgical and nephrology teams.

CONTRAINDICATIONS TO BECOMING A LIVING RENAL DONOR

The following situations will **prohibit a person from becoming a live donor:**

- Age younger than 18 or older than 65.
- These risks for developing renal disease:
  - o Glomerular filtration rate less than 80 ml/min.
  - o Hematuria or proteinuria.
  - o Structural abnormalities in the kidneys.
  - o History of recurrent nephrolithiasis (kidney stones).
- Comorbidities:
  - o COPD
  - o Diabetes
  - o Emotional instability
  - o Hypertension
  - o Hepatitis B or C
  - o HIV
  - o Mental instability

- o Substance abuse
- o Thromboembolic disease
- History of significant systemic disorders.
- Positive HLA crossmatch between donor and recipient.
- High surgical risk (bleeding disorders, arrhythmia, known adverse reactions to general anesthesia).

SURGICAL METHODS FOR LIVING DONOR NEPHRECTOMY

There are **three surgical methods** that can be used for a living donor nephrectomy: Open nephrectomy, laparoscopic nephrectomy, and hand-assisted laparoscopic nephrectomy. A hand-assisted laparoscopic nephrectomy is very similar to a laparoscopic nephrectomy. The patient is placed in a lateral decubitus position while the surgical table is flexed at midpoint to maximize the flank surface area. Carbon dioxide is used as an inflator to maximize visualization. Three to four abdominal incisions are made for a camera and surgical equipment. In a hand-assisted procedure, one of the abdominal incisions is used by the surgeon to place one hand inside of the Pneumo Sleeve. A Pneumo Sleeve is a device that maintains cavity inflation with carbon dioxide. While the Pneumo Sleeve maintains abdominal inflation, the surgeon retrieves the donor kidney with his or her hand. Once the kidney has been located the Pneumo Sleeve is inverted. The inverted sleeve forms a bag in which the kidney is placed.

OPEN NEPHRECTOMY AND LAPAROSCOPIC NEPHRECTOMY

For an **open nephrectomy**, place the patient in the lateral position with flexion to extend the surface of the flank area (between the ribs and the hips). The surgeon makes a flank incision right above or below the 11th or 12th rib. The surgeon may need to remove a rib portion. Take special care not to disturb the pleura and abdominal organs.

For a **laparoscopic nephrectomy**, place the patient lying in the lateral decubitus position with the surgical table flexed at midpoint to maximize the exposure of the flank area. Inflate the abdominal cavity with carbon dioxide for easier visualization. The surgeon incises three or four small ports on the outside of the abdomen. Place a video camera through the primary port. The surgeon uses the remaining ports as a passageway for surgical instruments. Once the surgeon has detached the kidney, it is removed through one of the small abdominal ports.

LAPAROSCOPIC NEPHRECTOMY: BENEFITS AND DISADVANTAGES

The benefits and disadvantages of a **laparoscopic nephrectomy versus an open nephrectomy**:

Traditional Open Nephrectomy	Laparoscopic Nephrectomy
Hospital stay of 2-4 days	Hospital stay of 1-2 days
O.R. time is 55-65 minutes	O.R. time is much longer, *unless the surgeon is very experienced*
Foot-long surgical incision with noticeable scar	3-4 small keyhole incisions with minimal scarring
Only 5% of patients require this approach	A laparoscopic nephrectomy costs about $2,000 more than an open nephrectomy, but it is more popular because there is less time off work, fewer drugs, and less pain.

DONOR NEPHRECTOMY

STANDARD OF CARE FOR DONOR POST-OPERATIVELY

The **post-operative donor nephrectomy patient** is sent to the post anesthetic care unit (PACU) for 1-2 hours. If the patient is intubated, the O.R. nurse assists the PACU nurse with extubation. The PACU nurse connects the patient to a heart monitor, pulse oximetry, and blood pressure monitor, and performs a quick assessment of the patient's breathing and circulatory status. Once the vital signs have been recorded, the O.R. nurse reports to the PACU nurse a comprehensive description of the surgical procedure, including:

- Any surgical difficulties that occurred in the OR
- IV fluids, blood products, and medications administered during surgery
- A list of invasive lines, drainage systems, intact gauzes, incisional care, and known drug sensitivities

The PACU nurse now performs a detailed assessment, and continues to monitor the donor's vital signs frequently.

POSSIBLE COMPLICATIONS ASSOCIATED WITH LIVING RENAL DONATION

Short-term complications associated with a living renal donation include: Atelectasis; pneumonia; pneumothorax; thromboses in the lungs; hypotension; urinary retention; urinary tract infection; wound complications; intestinal complications; injuries to the spleen; thrombophlebitis and deep vein thromboses (DVT). Most of these complications can be reversed soon after they materialize. The perioperative mortality rate for a living renal donor is very low, at 0.03%.

The **long-term risks** of being a living renal donor are also low. Most of the complications are associated with having only one kidney. Persons with one kidney are at greater risk of developing low-grade proteinuria. Renal donors are also at risk for higher serum creatinine levels, with a lower creatinine clearance. In spite of these findings, it does not increase their chances of developing high blood pressure.

INTERVENTIONS FOR COMPLICATIONS

Following a donor nephrectomy, complications may arise. The interventions are described below:

- **Atelectasis** is lung collapse. Initiate aggressive pulmonary toileting with an incentive spirometer. Encourage the patient to perform deep breathing exercises and coughing. Assist the patient to frequently change positions.
- **Hypoxia** is lack of oxygen from hypoventilation. Hypoxia is frequently observed immediately post op as the result of anesthesia and/or narcotic-induced respiratory depression. Decrease or discontinue the prescribed narcotic, and give Narcan if indicated. Lift up the head of the bed to at least 45 degrees to facilitate improved pulmonary expansion.
- **Fever** is usually related to lung collapse or a secondary infection. Obtain culture samples immediately and send them to the lab for sensitivity testing. Begin pulmonary toileting. Start antibiotic therapy as appropriate, and give antipyretics for comfort.
- **Hypotension** is usually related to a fluid imbalance, narcotic use, or bleeding. Rarely is sepsis the cause of low blood pressure. Begin IV fluids as per order. Monitor vital signs frequently until they stabilize. Consider the possible need for a blood transfusion or colloid.

- **Tachycardia** is a rapid heart rate (over 100 beats per minute), usually from a fluid imbalance, pain and anxiety. Even if the patient's heart rate does not exceed 100, if he or she complains of palpitations, treat him or her for tachycardia. Give IV fluids and pain medications per order. If an unstable rhythm is suspected (anything other than normal sinus rhythm), order an EKG immediately.
- If a **pneumothorax** is present, the surgeon may have unintentionally cut the pleura. Administer oxygen as ordered. Many times, a small pneumothorax will resolve without intervention. In more severe cases, a chest tube may be required to re-expand the pulmonary cavity.
- Frequently, **nausea and vomiting (n/v)** are associated with anesthesia or the use of narcotics. Keep the patient NPO (nothing by mouth). Give appropriate IV fluids and electrolytes. Administer anti-nausea medications, like Gravol suppositories. Once n/v subsides, slowly resume the patient's regular diet. In some instances, a nasogastric (NG) tube will need to be placed if the patient cannot eat.
- **Thrombophlebitis** is usually the result of being sedentary. The O.R. staff should apply antiembolism stockings and SCD to both legs, and these devices should remain in use until the patient is capable of getting up and walking independently. Anticoagulation with Coumadin or heparin may be required.
- **Wound infection** is almost always the result of a bacterial infection. Deferred healing and scarring can result in a hernia. Wound infections should be treated with organism-specific antibiotics. Consult a microbiologist.
- **Flatulence** (gas pain) **and constipation** result from heavy narcotic use, lack of mobility, and carbon dioxide gas used during laparoscopic procedures. Administer a stool softener for mild cases, and a laxative for moderate cases. Severe cases require an enema. Stress to the donor patient the importance of regular ambulation and adequate fluid intake.
- **Poor pain control** is from surgical incisions, lack of movement, and/or uneasiness. Change the patient's pain medication, strength, and route. Consult a pain management specialist.

DISCHARGE INSTRUCTIONS FOR POST-TRANSPLANT RENAL DONOR

Discharge instructions for the post-transplant renal donor include:

- Drink 8 glasses of fluid a day. Avoid coffee, tea, and cola.
- Eat frequent, small meals with protein (meat, eggs, peanut butter, legumes, and milk).
- Take pain medication and stool softeners for at least two weeks.
- Avoid activities that could injure remaining kidney.
- Don't lift over 10 pounds; avoid shoveling, raking, and vacuuming for 6 weeks. Do not drive for at least 3 weeks.
- Avoid returning to work for 4-8 weeks, or 12 weeks if your job involves lifting. (For women) Avoid pregnancy.
- Avoid bathtubs or swimming pools for 2 weeks (showers ok).
- Keep your follow-up appointments. Report these signs and symptoms *immediately*: Pus, drainage, redness, odor or swelling in your incision.
- Fever over 38°C or 104°F/Uncontrolled pain, or new onset of pain in the back/Lengthy bouts of nausea or vomiting/Difficulty urinating /Pain in the legs – DO NOT MASSAGE YOUR CALF
- Provide patient with list of contact numbers: Transplant center; physicians; transplant coordinators. Review discharge medications (name of medications, purpose, dosage, frequency, side effects).

- Show patient how to clean and dry the incision, and how to trim off the ends of the Steri-Strips after the first week. Tell patient to let the rest of the Steri-Strips drop off of their own accord.

VACCINES FOR KIDNEY TRANSPLANT RECIPIENTS

All kidney transplant recipients need to be **vaccinated** against influenza in mid-October every year, with the exception of those who have a known allergy to eggs or egg products. A transplant recipient should never be given a live vaccine, nor be exposed to the body fluids of someone who has recently received a live vaccine. Because the immune system of an organ recipient patient is in a suppressed state, exposure to the live vaccine could actually cause the active disease. Live vaccines to be avoided are:

- Bacille Calmette-Guerin (BCG).
- MMR (measles, mumps, and rubella).
- Oral polio vaccine (OPV).
- Typhoid, TY21a.
- Smallpox.
- Varicella (chicken pox).
- Yellow fever.

POST-OPERATIVE SEX AND PREGNANCY

ALL ADULT RECIPIENTS

Resume sexual activity when the incision has healed, and you and your partner feel comfortable with sex. Don't put pressure on the dialysis access site. If you have self-image issues because of surgical scars and drug side effects, we can arrange sex therapy. You may have had sexual problems before your surgery because of high blood pressure and anemia. Fertility and libido usually return to normal within a few weeks. Steroid side-effects, impotence, and vaginal dryness are certainly treatable.

TEENAGERS

Dialysis may have made the patient smaller than their peers, and less sexually mature. The transplant will help resolve these issues.

BANFF 97 GRADING SYSTEM FOR ACUTE REJECTION

The Banff 97 grading system rates the severity of an acute renal rejection episode, based on the microscopic findings of a tissue biopsy. Each tissue sample is rated from 1-3. The lower the grade number, the better. The degree of rejection is determined by the presence or absence of: Tubulitis (the presence of WBC's in the renal tubule epithelium); intimal arteritis; transmural inflammation; and fibrinoid necrosis. The Banff 97 grading system indicates the reversibility of the rejection episode, and suggests what treatment should be prescribed. If the patient is rated borderline to grade 2A-2B, IV Solu-Medrol is prescribed. If the patient has grades 2B-3B, then monoclonal antibodies (mAb or moAb), or polyclonal antibodies (Atgam or Thymoglobulin) derived from different B-cell lines are prescribed.

MEDICATION THERAPY TO TREAT MILD-TO-MODERATE ACUTE CELLULAR REJECTION

When **mild-to-moderate acute cellular rejection** is detected, the standard treatment by most physicians is 500 mg IV Methylprednisolone for 3 consecutive days. The dose is tapered down over the next 3 days to 250 mg, 75 mg, and 15 mg. After the six-day course of Methylprednisolone is complete, oral Prednisone is started at 60 mg/day for 2 days, 40 mg/day for 2 days, and 30 mg/day

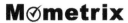

thereafter as the maintenance dose. High dose steroids tend to cause diabetogenic effects. For that reason, be sure to monitor glucose levels carefully on all high-dose steroid patients.

DRUG THERAPY TO TREAT MODERATE-TO-SEVERE ACUTE CELLULAR REJECTION

Drugs that treat **moderate-to-severe acute cellular rejection** are polyclonal antibodies or monoclonal antibodies, such as mAb or moAb. Examples of polyclonal antibodies are Atgam and Thymoglobulin. Muromonab CD3 is a monoclonal antibody. The polyclonal antibodies diminish lymphocytes that are circulating in the bloodstream, especially T-cells, which are responsible for cellular rejection. The polyclonal antibody of choice is Thymoglobulin because it has been found to be more effective, more likely to reverse rejection, and less costly than some alternative treatments. The standard dose for Thymoglobulin is 1.5 mg/kg. The dose for Atgam is 10-15 mg/kg. The usual dose for Muromonab is 5 mg IV push. However, if the patient does not show improvement after the 5 mg dose, it can be increased to 10 mg. The treatment course with antibodies is usually 7-14 days, depending on how quickly a response is seen.

THROMBOSES AND WOUND INFECTIONS

Thrombosis is a blood clot that stays in the artery or vein where it originated. Thrombosis happens because: The blood vessel was occluded from surgical trauma, technical problems occurred with the donor kidney, or cytokines were released from Muromonab-CD3 therapy. Suspect a major vessel thrombosis if the patient: Was producing an adequate urine flow, but it stopped abruptly or is slowly decreasing, has discomfort at the graft site, has a high creatinine level, and blood in the urine (hematuria). Ask the attending physician to order an EL test immediately to confirm the presence of a thrombosis and determine if the kidney is still viable. If the thrombus reduced the blood supply to the kidney and there is tissue necrosis, inform the surgeon and prep the patient for a transplant nephrectomy.

Wound infections result from immunosuppressive therapy, which increases the patient's susceptibility to infections. Diabetic patients are at greater risk of developing a post-transplant infection due to impeded healing time. Prophylactic cephalosporin is prescribed for the first 24 hours post-surgery.

ACUTE TUBULAR NECROSIS

Acute tubular necrosis (ATN) is death of the kidney tubule cells that transport urine to the ureters. ATN is characterized by cessation of urine output (anuria) or by scanty urine output (oliguria) ranging in duration from a few days to several weeks. The glomerular filtration rate (GFR) declines and BUN and creatinine levels rise. Known risk factors that contribute to ATN are: Ageing; cold ischemia time greater than 24 hours; hemodynamic instability pre-transplant; toxic reaction to the suspension used to flush the kidneys, and kidney sepsis from improper cleansing. ATN is treated with a monoclonal or polyclonal antibody. While antibody treatment is underway, withhold the calcineurin inhibitor, because it increases the patient's risk of nephrotoxicity. If ATN persists longer than a week post-transplant, suggest to the attending physician that a tissue biopsy should be performed, to rule out organ rejection.

LYMPHOCELES AND URINE LEAKS AS POST-RENAL TRANSPLANT COMPLICATIONS

A **lymphocele** is an accumulation of lymphatic fluid around the transplanted kidney because blood vessels were tied off poorly during surgery (ligation). Signs and symptoms of lymphoceles include: Frequency and urgency (urinating often and uncontrollably), pain and tenderness, and incontinence as a result of pressure from the lymphocele. The iliac vein can also develop an obstruction, resulting in swelling of the leg. Lymphoceles are diagnosed thorough an ultrasound.

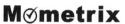

Urine leaks are due to a reconnection problem with the blood vessels serving the ureters and bladder, but can be mistaken for organ rejection. A yellow, serous drainage may be seen if the patient's urine output is acceptable. Collect a sample of the drainage for creatinine analysis. A significantly high creatinine level can indicate a urine leak. A small leak can be fixed by decompression of the bladder with a catheter. If the problem persists, surgery will be necessary.

BLEEDING AND RENAL ARTERY STENOSIS

Bleeding can occur during the first 24 hours after a renal transplant from anticoagulants (heparin), low clotting factors, or because vessels were not ligated or cauterized properly during the surgical procedure. Signs of internal bleeding include: Pallor; diaphoresis; cool, clammy skin; significant abdominal pain; swelling; tenderness or bruising; abnormal pulse; rapid breathing; and a steadily declining hematocrit level. Order an ultrasound or CT immediately if internal bleeding is suspected.

Renal artery stenosis is a narrowing or blockage of the artery that supplies blood to the kidney. Renal artery stenosis is generally seen a few months after transplantation, but does not exceed one year after the kidney transplant. The first signs of renal artery stenosis are usually uncontrolled high blood pressure and decreasing renal function. A bruit can be detected over the stenotic artery. The narrowing stenotic passage can be managed with angioplasty, but recurrent stenosis requires surgical intervention.

DEVELOPMENT OF HYPOPHOSPHATEMIA POST-RENAL TRANSPLANT

The four primary reasons **hypophosphatemia** develops are:

1. Elevated parathyroid hormone (PTH), which increases phosphate excretion via the kidneys.
2. Low vitamin D levels, which are generally the consequence of delayed or inadequate digestion of phosphate in the intestines.
3. Corticosteroid use, which diminishes tubular reuptake of phosphate.
4. Immunosuppressive therapy, which causes the proximal tubules to increase urinary excretion of phosphate.

If the transplant patient presents with hypophosphatemia, always verify first if they are still on a phosphate binder. K-Phos Neutral is a phosphate supplement that offers the greatest amount of phosphate with the smallest amount of potassium. Neutra Phos is an option, but has 7.13 mEq of potassium per dose, so has a high risk of hyperkalemia. Take great precautions to make sure the correct dose of phosphate is given.

CAUSE OF DEATH AFTER A RENAL TRANSPLANT

Post-renal transplantation, the most common **cause of death** is blood vessel disease, like heart attack (MI), stroke, and congestive heart failure. Diabetic and hypertensive patients are at increased risk for blood vessel disease. Immunosuppressants cause arteriosclerosis (hardening of the arteries) to develop, or if it already exists, to progress at a faster rate. Conduct a stringent preoperative assessment to detect underlying cardiovascular disease that may worsen due to complications from anesthesia, surgery, and immunosuppressive therapy. Pre-op diagnostic tests should include: An echocardiogram; cardiac stress test; cardiac catheterization; and carotid Doppler studies. Carefully monitor the patient for signs and symptoms of a thrombus (stationary blood clot) or embolus (traveling blood clot) after catheterization and surgery.

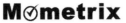

Pancreas Transplant

PROSPECTIVE RECIPIENTS

A **pancreas transplant** is typically reserved for patients who have already been diagnosed with Type I diabetes. On rare occasions, a patient may receive a pancreas transplant as a pre-emptive measure, to prevent him or her from developing diabetes. In the latter instance, the organ recipient requires a total pancreatectomy. Islet of Langerhans cells located in the pancreas are responsible for insulin production. Potential pancreas transplant patients have dysfunctional islet cells as a result of fever, disease or trauma, and make little or no insulin. Lack of insulin production by the pancreas leads to unregulated blood glucose levels. Type II diabetics are not usually considered eligible to receive a pancreas transplant, because they continue to produce insulin; however, the insulin is not able to regulate blood glucose levels adequately.

EVALUATION

All patients on an organ donation recipient list undergo the same routine tests. In addition to these, potential pancreas recipients must undergo an extensive cardiovascular assessment. Cardiovascular health is a major concern in a diabetic patient. Any patient over 45 year of age, or who has had diabetes for more than 20 years, must undergo a Doppler echocardiogram and cardiac stress test. If abnormalities are found, a heart catheterization and carotid arteries assessment for stenosis should follow. Other studies include: Nerve conduction tests (to establish baseline neuropathy); extensive eye exam (to rule out or conclude the presence of retinopathy); and metabolic studies (including Hemoglobin A_1C). Cardiovascular reevaluation should be repeated every 6 months to screen for cardiovascular disease progression. Eye exams should be done once a year. Hemoglobin A_1C should be drawn every 3 months at a minimum.

PLACEMENT OF ALLOGRAFT PANCREAS

The transplanted pancreas is usually **placed** intraperitoneally, because the peritoneum (membrane that lines the abdominal cavity) has an ample vascular blood supply that aids in the absorption of pancreatic excretions. For both pancreas (PA) and simultaneous pancreas-kidney (SPK) transplants, the organ is placed most often in the right iliac fossa. The left iliac fossa is kept open, in case a future SPK transplant is needed. If this were to happen, the second pancreas transplant would be placed opposite the first transplanted pancreas. The patient's native pancreas is left undisturbed in its natural anatomical place. Although the native pancreas is no longer capable of producing insulin, it still provides much-needed enzymes and provides exocrine functions. The new pancreas only has the job of producing insulin to stabilize blood glucose levels. The digestive enzymes the transplanted pancreas produces are disposed of using either enteric drainage or urinary drainage.

DEFINITIVELY IDENTIFYING ORGAN REJECTION

During **preliminary pancreatic rejection**, islet cells continue to produce insulin and blood glucose levels remain normal, so it is very difficult to identify graft rejection before it is too late for organ survival. Missing early signs of graft rejection can result in inflammation, fibrosis of the graft, and islet cell destruction. It is only during the time of cell destruction that blood glucose levels rise. *Once hyperglycemia is established, the rejection process is irreversible.* Because of the difficulty in recognizing rejection, pancreas recipients make up the lowest percentage of graft survival rates. A biopsy of the pancreatic head is the definitive diagnosis for organ rejection.

WHEN REJECTION CAN BE IDENTIFIED

With an SPK transplant recipient, the transplanted kidney is frequently the first to become involved in the rejection process. The first signs of kidney rejection are: A rapid increase in serum creatinine

47

levels; transplant site pain; and elevated temperature. A biopsy tissue sample must be taken before initiating treatment for organ rejection. If the biopsy sample confirms rejection, it is assumed that the recipient is rejecting both organs. However, SPK biopsies are so difficult that they are usually deferred until it is too late. As with pancreas transplants, SPK transplants do not produce elevated blood glucose levels until the pancreatic islet cells are already in the process of being destroyed.

ADVANTAGES AND DISADVANTAGES OF ENTERIC VERSUS URINARY DRAINAGE

Enteric drainage involves taking part of the donor's duodenum, along with the pancreas, and transplanting it in such a fashion that all enzymes are drained into the small bowel and excreted with the stool. **Urinary drainage** simply means draining the enzymes into the bladder, to be eliminated with urination. There remains controversy over which method is superior. Each method has its advantages and disadvantages. Enteric drainage offers less urinary tract infections, but comes with the risk factor of an anastomotic leak that can cause pancreatitis and/or sepsis. Urinary drainage has less risk factors, but does offer increased occurrence of frequent, severe urinary tract infections (UTI). 25% of all patients who opt for urinary drainage must convert to enteric drainage 6 months after a pancreas transplant because of severe urinary symptoms.

Liver Transplant

SCREENING TESTS

Screening tests for a liver transplant include the following:

Laboratory Medicine	Antimitochondrial antibody (AMA); antinuclear antibody (ANA); Chemistry A panel, including BUN, cholesterol, triglycerides, fasting blood sugar (FBS), liver enzymes, total protein, T_3, T_4, and TSH; CBC; PT/PTT; hepatitis; HIV; CMV; EBV; and prostate specific antigen (PSA)
Imaging	Colonoscopy; CT scan; endoscopy; multiple gated acquisition scan; Doppler4 ultrasound of the hepatic vein and artery
Pathology	Liver Biopsy
Cardiology	Angiogram/arteriogram, echocardiogram, EKG
Resp.	Pulmonary function tests
Gyn.	PAP smear, mammogram, pelvic exam
Urology	Prostate exam

PHYSIOLOGICAL FACTORS THAT LIMIT CHANCES OF RECEIVING TRANSPLANT

Patient is unlikely to receive a **liver** transplant:

- Alcohol or drug abuse/addiction
- Extrahepatic primary malignant neoplasms (EPMN)
- Elevated blood pressure in the lungs (pulmonary hypertension)
- Failure of 3 or more organ systems (multi-system organ failure)
- Severe cardiopulmonary disease

This list is not all-inclusive and does not imply a guarantee of organ rejection. However, these factors usually play a significant role in organ rejection, regardless of where the transplant center is located.

POSSIBLE DANGERS WITH LIVING LIVER DONOR PROCEDURE

Disclose all of the following **risks** to the potential donor and his or her family prior to liver surgery in language they can understand:

- External scarring.
- Post-operative pain.
- Infection.
- Sequellae associated with anesthesia, intubation, DVT, PE, cholecystectomy, and line placement.
- Possibility of liver failure (acute or chronic) requiring a liver transplant.
- Risk of blood or blood product-related reactions.
- Wound dehiscence, intestinal blockage, ileus, hernia, and adhesions, which may impact future abdominal surgeries.
- Significant, debilitating fatigue.
- Denial of health insurance coverage and future health care.

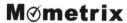
Explain to the potential donor and family the chances of mortality and morbidity. Provide them with written comparative data that includes statistics by center, nationally, and internationally.

PROCEDURE TO SURGICALLY REMOVE AND PRESERVE DONOR LIVER

The surgeon places a catheter into the donor's distal abdominal aorta and splenic vein branch of the inferior mesenteric vein. With the liver still attached to the donor, the perfusionist infuses it with a preservative solution to begin the cooling process that is obligatory to maintain organ viability. Once infusion is complete, the surgeon begins the removal process. Careful steps are taken to preserve the hepatic artery, portal vein, and common bile duct. Once the liver is removed, it is immediately packed in ice for transport to the recipient's hospital. Once removed from the donor, the liver will remain viable for 24 hours. However, most transplant centers strive for transplantation to occur within 12 hours, to reduce the risk of primary non-function, hepatic artery thrombosis, and biliary complications that occur if more than 12 hours elapses.

RESECTING THE LIVER

The surgeon must tailor a living liver division for each individual case, because livers differ. Every liver has two main sections—the right and left lobes. The left lobe makes up approximately 40% of the total liver volume. The right lobe makes up approximately 60% of the total liver volume. However, for functional purposes, the liver can be divided into eight different sections, corresponding with the bile duct system and blood supply furnished by the portal vein. Essentially, four different types of procedures can be performed to correctly resection the liver of a living donor:

- Left lateral segmentectomy
- Left lobectomy
- Right lobectomy
- Standard right lobe resection

LIVING DONOR PROCEDURES AND LIVER REGENERATION

Recipient size is a key factor in the surgeon's choice of which living donor procedure to use. For pediatric living donor transplantation, the left lateral segment of the liver is used. This segment of the liver can also be used in adolescents and some smaller adults. The right lobe of the liver is used for most adult-to-adult living liver transplants. The transplant team realizes that the more liver volume they remove, the greater the risk to the donor. The liver does have the capacity to regenerate itself. The regeneration process begins immediately after liver division and transplantation, and can continue for up to one year post operatively. The recipient graft and remaining donor liver will grow to reach a normal volume for each individual.

MINIMUM FUNCTIONAL LIVER GRAFT

Several formulae are available to help the surgeon calculate the **minimum volume of functional liver graft** required to support all of the recipient's metabolic needs. The most popular formula involves body surface area:

$$\text{Standard liver volume (ml)} + 706.2 \times (\text{body surface area [M2]}) + 2.4$$

Using this formula, one study found that good recipient outcomes were based on a GV/SV range from 31-54%. Although this is the most common formula, in some circumstances the surgeon may choose a formula that calculates the graft weight versus the recipient's body weight ratio (GRWR), or graft-to-recipient body ratio (GRBW). However, the graft survival rate when using these formulae is much lower. Other factors that adversely affect the outcome of a living donor liver transplant (LDLTx) are portal vein thrombosis, obesity, marginal psychosocial function, and re-transplantation.

POST-TRANSPLANT FOLLOW-UP TESTS FOR LIVER RECIPIENT

Initially, it is mandatory for a liver recipient to have blood tests drawn every 2-3 weeks post-transplant. If the liver functions well, and immunosuppressive therapy is well regulated, then blood tests decrease to once every 3 months. Each transplant center has its own protocol. At the one-year anniversary of the transplant, these tests are recommended for both genders:

- Ultrasound of the liver to check for vessel patency.
- Bone density test.
- Chest x-ray.
- Bloodwork for cholesterol, triglyceride, uric acid, Hemoglobin A_1C, and Hepatitis B and C screening.
- Dental exam.
- Eye exam.
- Skin cancer screening.
- 24-hour urine test.

Additional tests for women are a mammogram and Pap smear. Additional tests for men are a prostate exam and PSA test.

MONITORING A NEWLY TRANSPLANTED LIVER

The **monitoring of a newly transplanted liver** starts in the Operating Room. These are all excellent indicators of the liver's functional level: Adequate kidney function; pH balance; coagulation normalization; body temperature stability; blood glucose levels; bile production; liver color; and hemodynamic stability. If the liver is not functioning properly, the exact cause must be identified quickly. Primary non-function requires a re-transplant almost immediately. Liver graft dysfunction can range from mild to severe, and may require supportive medical measures, but not necessarily re-transplantation. Other causes of liver dysfunction include thromboses (in the hepatic artery, portal vein, hepatic vein, or cavae), and biliary tract obstructions or leaks.

MICROCHIMERISM AND CHIMERISM

Microchimerism is the integration of donor and recipient cells, which occurs within minutes of a successful organ transplantation, once revascularization has been established. Over time, microchimerism may lead to immunologic non-reactivity and cell tolerance. The patient would no longer need immunosuppressive therapy. Tolerance is a drug-free state that has been successfully attained in some liver organ recipients. However, presently the only method to test tolerance is through trial and error. **Chimerism** is the combination of two incompatible parts to make a whole, which means the recipient must always be immunosuppressed to prevent organ rejection. Once a person receives a transplant, he or she is considered to be either chimeric or microchimeric.

STANDARD FOLLOW-UP PROTOCOL FOR LIVING LIVER DONORS

Most transplant centers require the liver donor to attend a **follow-up** visit one week after the donation. The doctor and donor discuss pain management, overall recovery status, and staple removal. The doctor checks the surgical wound for signs of infection. Visits continue once or twice a week, depending on the donor's symptoms. Medical Imaging will view the remaining liver within 3 months of surgery, using an MRI or CT scan. The purpose of the imaging is to evaluate the volumetric regeneration of the liver. At all follow-up visits, blood is drawn for liver function tests (LFT), a complete blood count (CBC), and chemistry. The donor's primary care physician should conduct an annual physical and report any abnormalities immediately to the transplant center. *The standard of care for long term follow-up of liver donors is still in debate.* This is a reasonable guideline only. Check the policy and procedure manual at the facility.

BILE LEAK IN LIVING DONOR

The classic signs and symptoms of a **bile leak** are: New onset fever; leukocytosis; abdominal pain; and persistent or increased bile leakage from the surgical drain. If the patient presents with these signs and symptoms, rule out a bile leak with medical imaging. Other potential reasons for these signs and symptoms are a biloma formation, or unspecified intra-abdominal collections. The liver's surface is the commonest site for a bile leak. Conservative treatment for a bile leak is to use the drainage tube that was previously placed during surgery. Usually, the bile leak will heal itself and will not require any form of surgical intervention. If the cause of the leak is traced back to a biloma or abscess, percutaneous drainage may be needed. The drain can be removed once the presence of bile subsides.

COMPLICATIONS THE LIVING LIVER DONOR MAY EXPERIENCE

Expect a living donor to have extreme fatigue, to the point of debilitation, for about the first month following surgery. A wound infection, although uncommon, is possible. Properly educate the donor about the signs and symptoms associated with infection. These minor gastrointestinal symptoms are also common for the first few weeks following surgery: Dyspepsia; early satiety; flatulence and bloating; constipation; and frequent bowel movements. Although their cause is not well understood, GI symptoms may result from gall bladder removal, colon manipulation, or from torsion of the remaining portion of the liver. Numbness below the surgical incision or abdominal tightness is also common after surgery. However, these symptoms should disappear within 3 months after surgery.

POST-OPERATIVE LIVER REJECTION

Liver rejection is when the organ recipient's body detects the allograft as non-self and initiates an immune system attack. Only 30% of liver transplant recipients are fortunate enough to avoid at least one episode of rejection. Typically, liver rejection occurs between 4-14 days post operatively. *If detected early, most episodes of liver rejection are reversible.* It is imperative that the recipient complies with all scheduled laboratory tests for liver enzymes, and reports these signs and symptoms of rejection: Tiredness; fever; jaundice; ascites; pain over the liver; pruritus; and dark-colored urine. The hepatologist will confirm suspicions of rejection by histopathologic verification with the Banff scale.

HEPATIC ENCEPHALOPATHY

Hepatic encephalopathy is neuropsychiatric changes in the patient's mental status due to advanced liver disease. The damaged liver cannot properly filter toxins, which begin to build up in the blood, causing confusion, disorientation, and insomnia. The grading system used to define the extent of the liver damage is mild, moderate, or severe. Encephalopathy is generally reversible through proper treatment of the precipitating factors. Dietary adjustments may be necessary, such as:

- Switching to a synthetic sugar or lactulose
- Eating a protein-restricted diet
- Using a nasogastric (NG) or endotracheal tube to avoid the danger of aspiration

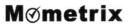

SPONTANEOUS BACTERIAL PERITONITIS AND HEPATORENAL SYNDROME

Spontaneous bacterial peritonitis (SBP) is inflammation of the peritoneum (lining of the abdomen), usually from enteric organisms in the ascitic fluid. Causes include: Cirrhosis of the liver; infected dialysis fluid; abdominal edema (ascites) associated with end-stage liver disease; and lupus or nephrosis in children. Whatever the cause of SBP, the prognosis is poor because it can result in decompensation of the liver. 30% of patients have no symptoms. Signs and symptoms include: Encephalopathy; diarrhea; ascites that does not improve with diuretics; renal failure; ileus; fever; chills; nausea; vomiting; hypotension; jaundice; and general malaise. Diagnosis is via paracentesis to collect ascitic fluid from the abdominal cavity. SBP is treated with antibiotics. *SBP is a contraindication for transplantation.*

Hepatorenal syndrome is a severe complication of cirrhosis and other liver diseases. Kidney dysfunction is caused by abnormalities in arterial circulation (vasoconstriction). The result of hepatorenal syndrome is **hyponatremia** that does not respond to an increase in fluids. Hepatorenal syndrome is usually reversible by transplantation.

HYPERLIPIDEMIA

Hyperlipidemia means excess lipids (fats) in the bloodstream, which leads to hardening of the arteries and cardiovascular disease. Up to 40% of all liver recipients develop high blood cholesterol levels (hypercholesterolemia). Risk factors for hyperlipidemia include:

- Cyclosporin instead of tacrolimus immunosuppressive therapy.
- Female gender.
- Cholestatic liver disease (e.g., gall stones, atresia, biliary cirrhosis).
- 3 boluses of steroids for rejection episodes.
- High pre-transplant cholesterol level (over 141 mg/dl).

Patients with hyperlipidemia (high fat levels in the blood) often develop xanthomas, small yellow nodules below their eyes, on their knees and elbows, and tendons. A white ring may appear around the eye. Hyperlipidemic patients complain of pain in the upper abdomen. The liver and spleen are tender to palpation, and the abdomen is swollen. Patients of any age can develop hyperlipidemia; it is not confined to older adults. If the patient has a total cholesterol level of 3.2 mmol/L or 240 mg/dl or above, this should be a sign for concern. Hyperlipidemia can be from:

- Diabetes
- Heredity (especially in French Canadians)
- Poor diet
- Iatrogenesis (drug-induced by cyclosporin and steroids)
- Chronic stress and smoking

DEVELOPMENT OF HYPERTENSION AFTER LIVER TRANSPLANT

Current statistics indicate that only 30% of all liver transplant recipients will avoid developing **high blood pressure** post operatively. The high prevalence is due to the use of corticosteroids and calcineurin inhibitors. The best way to lower blood pressure is to slowly decrease the dose of corticosteroids, or completely eliminate the corticosteroids from the medication regimen. Alternatively, decrease the calcineurin inhibitors, with or without the use of a calcineurin-sparing agent. Examples of calcineurin sparing agents are: Imuran, mycophenolate mofetil, and rapamycin.

Intestinal Transplant

PRELIMINARY EVALUATION

Each transplant center has its own evaluation process. Medical consults are determined based on each individual's diagnosis. Consult the facility's policies and procedures manual. Usually, the **intestinal transplant evaluation** is conducted over 3-5 days on an in-patient basis. Some centers have an out-patient evaluation process. The most common consults scheduled are: Gastroenterology; Cardiology; Pulmonary; Neurology; Psychiatry; Nutrition; Occupational Therapy; Physiotherapy; a multidisciplinary psychosocial assessment to evaluate the family support system, coping ability, medical compliance, and awareness of the disease and what the transplant process entails; and a child development specialist if the patient is under 18. The case manager responsible for co-coordinating all the consults, compiling their reports for the transplant team to review, and flagging any exclusionary factors.

PROCEDURES

The surgical team determines the type of transplant procedure to be performed based on the indication for the transplant, as well as other affected organs. The 3 types of intestinal transplant procedures are:

- **Isolated intestinal procedure:** Only the diseased portion of the small intestine is removed and replaced with a section of health donor intestine.
- **Composite graft**: The surgeon makes an enterectomy (removal and resection of part of the intestines) and hepatectomy (removal of all or part of the liver). Composite graft surgery is used for patients with short gut syndrome and TPN-induced cholestasis.
- **Multivisceral transplant:** Several different organ systems are involved in the surgical intervention. A multivisceral transplant can involve an enterectomy, gastrectomy, nephrectomy (removal of kidney) and/or pancreatectomy (removal of pancreas).

NUTRITIONAL NEEDS OF POST-TRANSPLANT PATIENT

Calorie intake is individually tailored to meet the requirements of each intestinal recipient. Factors to consider are: The patient's age; renal function; diabetic complications; number and type of rejection episodes; surgical re-explorations; infections; pancreatitis, and growth failure. Zinc levels are typically low during the first year post-transplant, due to high stomal outputs. Give the patient 1.5-3 times the RDA of zinc, and check zinc and albumin blood levels monthly. Continue the high doses of zinc until the patient's ostomy closes. Intestinal post-transplant recipients often have low folate and copper and require these as supplements. Give L-glutamine as an additive to enteral feedings. Glutamine is correlated with an increase in villous height and surface area, mucosal weight, and brush border enzyme activity. The recommended children's dose is 0.6 gm/kg/day, and for adults 30 gm/day.

DETERMINATION OF PROPER NUTRITIONAL ABSORPTION

Two significant indicators of proper graft function post-transplantation are sufficient **absorption** and **tolerance of feedings**. Evaluate these two indicators by measuring daily stomal outputs, serum electrolytes, nutritional markers, and note the incidence of blood or food particles in the stool. Assess carbohydrate absorption though a D-xylose breathalyzer test and the presence of fecal reducing substances. Improper absorption of fats is common among intestinal recipients and may be the result of the disturbance of the lymphatic system during surgery. A 24-hour stool collection measures the percentage of fat absorption and the level of fat-soluble vitamins present in the feces. Average stomal output should range from 40-60 m/kg/day in children, and 1-2 L/day in adults. Tacrolimus levels must be stable and satisfactory for adequate absorption. Increase the patient's fat

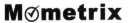

absorption and reduce stomal output by giving him or her: Pancreatic enzymes; a fat-soluble multivitamin daily; a low-fat diet; and interim IV intralipids.

ENTERAL FEEDING

Most **enteral feedings** are administered in the jejunostomy tube (JT) for 14 days post operatively if there are no problems. Enteral feedings are age-specific. Most consist of a low-osmolality, isotonic dipeptide formula with medium-chain triglycerides and glutamine, to allow for peak nutritional assimilation, nitrogen use, and fat uptake, while avoiding hyperosmolar diarrhea. The typical JT feeding is administered on a continuous basis at a low rate. The standard starting dose is 2 ml/hr for infants and 10 ml/hr for adults. The dosage can gradually be increased until caloric requirements are acquired as the TPN is decreased. Once the goal rate is reached, the strength is gradually increased until full strength is tolerated.

RADIOALLERGOSORBENT TESTING

Radioallergosorbent test (RAST): A blood test for Allergen-specific Immunoglobulin E (IgE), which determines the patient's food allergies or causes of asthma. RAST is used instead of skin pricking and inhalation tests when the patient is taking antihistamines or has dermatitis. 130 ng/ml is high normal. *RAST may give false-negative results if the allergen is cooked or processed.* Order IgG with RAST to get a clear result. Lactose and gluten are two common food allergies among intestinal transplant recipients. Enteral feeding supplements are necessary for the intestinal recipient for the first few months post op, until the patient's ability to meet caloric requirements orally is firmly established.

Factors that affect oral intake in *all* patients	Special factors that affect oral intake in *children*:
GERD with aspiration Hypergag reflex Hospital environment Behavioral issues	Limited feeding experience Parenting factors Developmental delays Need for special assistance from Occupational Therapy and Speech

DETECTION OF INTESTINAL GRAFT REJECTION EPISODES

A **surveillance endoscopy** is conducted through the ileostomy twice a week for the first 4-6 weeks post-transplantation. The gap between endoscopies progressively increases, providing the recipient's clinical status is stable, and taking into account the recipient's rejection history and risk factors for rejection. After 3 years post-transplant, most intestinal transplant recipients are scheduled only once a year for a follow-up endoscopy. The physician performing the endoscopy looks closely at the intestinal mucosa to see if it has a normal pink, velvety appearance from healthy villi. Clinical indicators of rejection are edema, granularity, erythema (redness), and duskiness (blue cyanosis). If rejection is well advanced, frail tissue with scattered ulcerations can be identified. Severe rejection findings include mucosal ulcers, aperistalsis (absent peristalsis with lack of bowel sounds), and denuded mucosa with pseudomembranes. A definitive diagnosis of intestinal rejection requires a Histology report.

ALLOGRAFT REJECTION

Currently, the overall incidence of **intestinal transplant rejection** is 90%, because there is a large amount of lymphoid tissue linked to the intestines. Intestinal rejection is most frequently seen during the first six months post-transplant. Nevertheless, intestinal rejection can occur at any time. Isolated intestinal recipients have the greatest occurrence of rejection (88%), and the most severe symptoms. Composite liver-intestine grafts have a 66% rejection rate. Multivisceral grafts have a 75% rejection rate. Because the liver is rejected in 43% of cases where it was a composite graft with the intestine, researchers think the liver may play a defensive role whenever it is a component of a composite graft.

CHRONIC, ACUTE, AND SEVERE INTESTINAL REJECTION

Chronic intestinal transplant rejection develops over an extended time period through repetitive acute rejection episodes that are incompletely resolved or resistant to treatment. In **acute intestinal transplant rejection,** HLA antibodies develop after transplantation, with abrupt onset of illness that progresses quickly. **Severe intestinal transplant rejection** mostly affects the ileum and requires aggressive immunosuppression with antilymphocyte serum to prevent concomitant kidney and renal failure.

WARNING SIGNS OF ACUTE REJECTION

Currently, there are no specific serum tests that can detect rejection in intestinal transplant patients. Researchers are focusing on serum citrulline, a nonessential amino acid produced by the mucosa of the intestines, as a likely marker for intestinal rejection. The most reliable way to detect an intestinal graft rejection is through clinical assessment, endoscopic finding, and histologic conclusions. Intestinal rejection can vary from mild to severe. Sepsis often goes together with rejection, due to bacterial or fungal translocation secondary to the disturbance of the mucosal barrier of the intestine. Severe rejection can have the devastating consequences of graft enterectomy or death. The most common **clinical symptoms of acute rejection are:**

- Noticeable variation in stool output
- Elevated temperature
- Malaise
- Abdominal pain and distention
- Nausea/vomiting
- Dusky stoma
- GI bleeding*
- Ileus*
- Septic shock syndrome*
- Acute respiratory distress syndrome*

*Symptoms of severe rejection.

INTESTINAL REJECTION TREATMENT

Mild-to-moderate and severe intestinal rejection is treated:

Mild-to-moderate	Severe
Increase the tacrolimus dose to 20-25 ng/ml. Give IV bolus Methylprednisolone with decreasing cycled doses over 5 days. Adjunctive therapy may also be initiated. Endoscopy with biopsy is performed twice a week.	Give Muromonab-CD3 for up to 14 days; exact treatment length depends on biopsy findings. Rabbit Antithymocyte Globulin is currently used in some institutions over Muromonab-CD3.

PRIMARY MEDICAL CONCERNS IN POST-TRANSPLANT RECIPIENT

Aside from graft rejection, **fluid and electrolyte balance** are concerns during the early post-operative period. Patients commonly develop intravascular volume depletion while concurrently retaining fluid shortly after transplant. The cause for this may be due to an increase in interstitial fluid accumulation in the peripheral tissue, the intestinal graft, and the lungs in the presence of escalating ascites from leakage of mesenteric lymphatics. Pay special attention to kidney function and electrolytes. Keep strict I & O measurements for exact adjustments in IV fluids. Typically, fluids are administered at two-thirds maintenance to sustain a central venous pressure of 6-10 cm H_2O and a urinary output of 0.5-1.5 ml/kg/hr. Fluid imbalances result from an increased stomal output of water, sodium, magnesium, and bicarbonate. The long-term goal is for all intestinal transplant recipients to be able to tolerate a regular oral diet without supplemental support by one year post operatively for adults, and two years post operatively for children.

INTESTINAL TRANSPLANT COMPLICATIONS

The following are **three intestinal transplant complications**:

- **Gastrointestinal bleeding:** GI bleeding results from rejection or infection, and is the most frequent hurdle to overcome following an intestinal transplant. An endoscopy with biopsy must be performed immediately for a differential diagnosis. Aggressive medical treatment must be started as soon as possible to avoid surgery.
- **Leaks:** Poor surgical technique or delayed wound healing around the gastrointestinal vessels where they were re-connected can result in leaks during the first week post-transplant. However, medical advancements have lessened the risk of intestinal leaks through decompression by jejunostomy and ileostomy.
- **Hypermotility:** The GI peristalsis of the intestinal graft is altered, causing diarrhea throughout the early postoperative period. Antidiarrheal medications and a high fiber diet used in combination are usually enough to control the symptoms of hypermotility. However, hypermotility can also be a sign of allograft rejection or surgical contamination, so the cause of hypermotility must always be established. If hypermotility is present, take the patient's temperature and observe the abdomen for swelling. Report fever and distention to the attending physician immediately.

INTESTINAL TRANSPLANT INFECTIONS

Over 80% of all intestinal transplant recipients will develop a bacterial infection, particularly Staphylococcus and Enterococcus. Enteric organisms are frequently discovered in abdominal incisions, pus-filled abdominal abscesses, infected peritonea, and pneumonia. Patients are placed on polymicrobial therapy to fight off multiple co-infections. If the patient has a fever and no apparent cause of infection can be identified, an endoscopy with tissue biopsy is performed. Although procedures vary by transplant center, prophylactic antibiotics are usually given for a maximum of 5 days post operatively.

Bacterial translocation can be prevented through selective bowel decontamination with enteral Tobramycin, colistimethate, and Amphotericin B for up to 2 weeks post-transplant. Take routine stool samples on all of intestinal transplant patients. If a culture reveals more than 10^8 organisms, the patient has sepsis or rejection. Notify the doctor on-call STAT, who will choose the most appropriate IV antibiotics to initiate, based on the sensitivity report from the Microbiology lab.

CYTOMEGALOVIRUS

Cytomegalovirus (CMV) is the most common viral infection among intestinal transplant recipients, occurring in 34% of all cases. CMV usually presents within the first six months following transplantation. Signs and symptoms include: Fever; gastroenteritis; muscular pain; joint pain; malaise; decreased appetite; focal ulcerations of the intestines accompanied by bleeding; leukopenia; thrombocytopenia; and atypical lymphocytosis. More often than not, CMV presents in the transplanted intestine. However, CMV can also cause: Gastroduodenitis; colitis of the native large intestine; pneumonitis; central nervous system disease; hepatitis; and retinitis. When the patient is febrile (fever is present), a standard work-up is completed with cultures of the urine, blood, stool, and sputum. If the patient is CMV-positive, his or her blood work will signify abundant CMV-inclusion bodies with inflammatory alterations. Endoscopy and histology exams confirm the CMV diagnosis.

FUNGAL INFECTIONS

The risk factors that predispose intestinal transplant recipients **to fungal infections** are:

- Health status before transplantation
- Large doses of immunosuppressants
- Intestinal leaks
- Surgical complications
- Extensive use of antibiotics
- IV contamination

Patients deemed to be at risk of developing a fungal infection are started on low-dose IV Amphotericin B prophylactically. Nystatin swish and swallow is used to prevent **candidiasis** (thrush) during high-dose immunosuppression. If refractory candidiasis is present, IV Amphotericin B or Fluconazole can be administered. If Fluconazole is started, monitor the patient for elevated tacrolimus levels, because the two drugs potentiate each other. If a systemic candida infection is present, it should be treated with IV Amphotericin B, Abelcet, or Fluconazole.

Transplantation Management

Evaluating Graft Function

GRAFT EVALUATION FOR FUNCTION

Elements of a **graft evaluation for function** may vary somewhat depending on the type of transplantation but generally includes:

- Assessing whether the organ appears to function as intended; for example, the heart beats, lungs inflate and deflate, and kidney produces urine.
- Carrying out baseline studies immediately post-transplantation to utilize as references.
- Assessing whether the apparent function is supported by laboratory findings and imaging (such as ultrasound or renal scintigraphy to assess flow of blood and function of transplanted kidney).
- Monitoring function of the transplanted organ for consistency over time, as deterioration may indicate graft failure.
- Monitoring temperature and vital signs for signs of deterioration and/or infection.
- Assessing patient's general feelings of well-being, energy level, appetite, mental status, and fecal and urinary output.
- Assessing changes in the patient's Karnofsky Status Scale (KPS) score and functional abilities, including ability to manage ADLs and mobility status.

GRAFT REJECTION

KIDNEY AND PANCREAS

Signs of **kidney graft rejection** include weight increase, increased BUN and creatinine, oliguria, peripheral edema, and fever as well as general malaise and fatigue and increased pain at operative site. Rejection is classified as hyperacute, accelerated, acute, and chronic, based on etiology, T-lymphocyte (most common) or B-lymphocyte mediated, and onset of symptoms:

- Hyperacute: Immediately after surgery.
- Accelerated: 24 hours to 5 days after surgery.
- Acute: A few days to weeks after surgery.
- Chronic: Months to years after surgery.

Initial signs of **pancreas graft rejection** in a patient who received a pancreas transplant with a bladder-drained graft include pain in right upper abdomen, increased serum amylase, and decreased urine amylase. Patients may develop flu-like symptoms, peripheral edema, and dyspnea. Symptoms are often very non-specific although hyperglycemia is usually a late sign as glucose levels remain within normal limits initially.

HEART AND LUNG

Signs of **heart graft rejection** include increased weakness, dyspnea, fever and/or chills, tachycardia, hypotension, peripheral edema, weight increase, decreased urinary output, poor appetite, nausea, and flu-like symptoms. Risk of rejection is greatest several weeks after surgery. Acute cellular rejection occurs when T-cell antibodies attack cardiac cells, usually within 3 to 6 months of transplantation. Humoral rejection may occur within the first 4 weeks or months or even years later. With humoral rejection, antibodies attack coronary arteries and other blood vessels. Chronic rejection, such as coronary artery vasculopathy impairs circulation to the heart muscle and may be asymptomatic until advanced.

Signs of **lung graft rejection** include increasing dyspnea and cough, flu-like symptoms, pulmonary congestion, fever and/or chills. Some patients, however, are essentially asymptomatic initially and identified through lung function testing. Cellular rejection (most common early) involves T-lymphocytes attacking lung tissue. Antibody-mediated rejection involves B-lymphocytes attacking the lung tissue. Acute rejection develops during the first 12 months and occurs in about 33% of lung transplant recipients. Chronic lung allograft dysfunction can include bronchiolitis obliterans syndrome, which leads to loss of the graft and/or death.

SMALL INTESTINE AND LIVER

Small intestine graft rejection is common because about 80% of immune cells are located within the small intestines. The section most at risk is the ileal portion of the bowel. Additionally, transplantation is associated with increased incidence of inflammatory bowel disease, putting the graft at risk. Antibody-mediated rejection is an ongoing concern. Acute graft rejection usually occurs within 90 days but can occur after 12 months. Patients may exhibit diarrhea, nausea and vomiting, abdominal pain, abdominal distention, and fever. Acute rejection is classified as indeterminate, mild, moderate, or severe. Chronic graft rejection may develop insidiously and patients may exhibit loss of weight, abdominal pain, and watery diarrhea. Chronic graft rejection often results in loss of the graft.

Signs and symptoms of **liver graft rejection** include increased bilirubin and jaundice, increased transaminase, dark-colored urine, pruritis, abdominal pain and distention, flu-like symptoms, dyspnea, cough, and nausea. Between 25 and 50 percent of recipients experience acute cellular rejection within the first 12 months, with risk the highest between weeks 4 and 6. Repeated episodes of acute cellular rejection may lead to chronic rejection, which may result in loss of the graft.

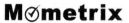

Signs and Symptoms of Rejection

TRANSPLANT RECIPIENT'S RISK OF INFECTION

The three factors that determine the transplant recipient's **risk for infection** are:

- Exposure to the public and hospital exposure (epidemiological).
- Current antibiotic regimen.
- Net degree of immunosuppression.

The two chief **types of infection exposure** within the hospital setting are domiciliary and nondomiciliary.

- **Domiciliary exposure** is coming in contact with infectious agents that reside on the patient's home unit. Examples of domiciliary exposure include air and water contamination. The pathogens that are often times responsible for domiciliary contamination include *Pseudomonas aeruginosa*, Vancomycin-resistant *Enterococcus faecium*, MRSA, and *Clostridium difficile*.
- **Nondomiciliary exposure** is contact with infectious agents that reside outside of the patient's unit. This type of exposure most commonly occurs during transport from one area to the next for tests or surgery.

IDENTIFYING INFECTION TRANSPLANT RECIPIENTS

Conventional x-rays are indispensable for diagnosing infections of the chest and central nervous system, the two most widespread and life-threatening causes of infections in transplant recipients. Single-lung transplant recipients can have abnormalities of the native lung that make diagnosing infection more complex. Look for the onset of new infiltrates. Depressed inflammatory response can greatly change the look of pulmonary lesions on the chest x-ray, or delay their appearance.

CT scans with or without contrast: can often give more accurate information than conventional x-rays. CT scans are preferred:

- When attempting to establish the degree of infection
- To follow a patient's reaction to treatment
- For pulmonary infections due to fungi or *Nocardia*
- For deciding which invasive diagnostic procedure should be used to collect microbiology and biopsy specimens
- For patients with frequent respiratory infections, to help identify secondary causative agents

COMMON INFECTIONS IN TRANSPLANT CANDIDATES

Transplant **candidates** can have asymptomatic infections that they do not know exist, e.g., from indwelling catheters or infected CPAP equipment. The transplant candidate's infection(s) go unnoticed until the stress of surgery, combined with immunosuppression, make them symptomatic or reactivate dormant infections, like herpes. Examples of **preexisting active infections**, divided by transplant type, are:

- **Kidney:** Unknown abscesses in the native kidneys; dialysis graft infections; peritoneal infections from contaminated dialysis fluid; and urinary tract infections (cystitis, pyelo).
- **Pancreas:** Kidney infections, especially for the female population.

- **Liver:** Intra-abdominal infections; aspiration pneumonia; and infections related to urinary catheter placement.
- **Heart:** Infections associated with catheter and pacemaker placement; and pneumonia.
- **Lung:** Pneumonia; pulmonary bacterial or fungal colonization.

COMMON POST-TRANSPLANTATION INFECTIONS

The type of infections that are more common at one month, 2-6 months, and more than six months post-transplantation:

Time Period	Type of Infection	Example
First month	Earl reactive or latent viruses	Herpes simplex virus reactivation; Human Herpes Virus 6
	Allograft infection transmitted from the donor	*Toxoplasma gondii* (in heart allograft); *Candida* supp. (from Trachea allograft in lung transplants)
2-6 months	Opportunistic organisms and viruses that modify the functioning of the immune system	Cytomegalovirus Epstein Barr virus *Pneumocystis carinii* *Listeria monocytogenes*
6+ months	Infections obtained as a result of public exposure	Upper respiratory tract infections (flu, adenoviruses)

VIRAL INFECTIONS

The most common post-transplant viral infections are discussed below:

- **Influenza virus:** Flu syndrome with secondary bacterial complications **Cytomegalovirus (CMV):** Pneumonitis, myocarditis, gastroenteritis, and rarely, pancreatitis, encephalitis, and retinitis **Papovavirus (HPV, SV40, BK, and JC):** Cancer, progressive multifocal leukoencephalopathy (PML), severe refractory anemia, fibrosing cholestatic hepatitis, pancytopenia, and thrombotic microangiopathy **Epstein-Barr virus (EBV):** Mononucleosis or post-transplant lymphoproliferative disease (PTLD), with nodal or extranodal effects on the Central Nervous System (CNS), gastrointestinal tract, lungs or bone marrow.
- **Herpes simplex 1 and 2 virus (HSV-1 and HSV-2):** Herpes labialis, herpetic esophagitis, anogenital lesions, and rarely, visceral infection **Varicella zoster virus:** Shingles or chickenpox.
- **Respiratory syncytial virus (RSV):** Bronchiolitis, nosocomial pneumonia, upper respiratory infection, lower respiratory tract disease, and organ rejection **Hepatitis virus:** Acute or chronic hepatitis, often with cirrhosis **Human herpes virus Type 6 (HHV-6):** Usually the A variant affects hematopoietic stem cell transplant recipients with bone marrow suppression, delayed engraftment, rash, fever, idiopathic pneumonitis, encephalitis, reactivated CMV, hepatitis, and graft-versus-host disease.

CMV

Cytomegalovirus (CMV) is the most widespread and significant pathogen for transplant recipients. 30-70% of all solid organ transplant recipients develop a CMV infection. Half of those infected experience symptoms of inflammation, tissue injury, opportunistic superinfections, allograft injury, and organ rejection. Native organs are not as susceptible to CMV as allograft organs are. Allograft outcomes are as follows:

- Kidney: Glomerulopathy
- Liver: Vanishing bile duct syndrome
- Heart: Accelerated cardiac vasculopathy
- Lung: Bronchiolitis obliterans

FUNGAL INFECTIONS

Fungal infections are less frequent than bacterial or viral infections in post-transplant recipients, but fungal infections have the highest mortality rate of the three types of infection. The three most common opportunistic fungi are *Candida, Cryptococci,* and *Aspergillus.* At present, the mortality rates for these three pathogens are: Candidiasis 23-71%; cryptococcosis 0-60%; and aspergillosis 20-100%. *Pneumocystis carinii* (PCP) was originally considered a protozoan. It has been renamed *Pneumocystis jiroveci* and reclassified as a fungal pathogen. The incidence of Pneumocystis pneumonia can be greatly reduced with prophylactic Trimethoprim/sulfamethoxazole. Antimicrobials that prevent and treat other fungal infections include Fluconazole, Amphotericin B, and Amphotericin B lipid complex. Oral thrust is treated with Nystatin and Clotrimazole troches (lozenges).

PARASITIC PATHOGENS IN TRANSPLANT RECIPIENTS

Cryptosporidium, Strongyloides stercoralis, and Toxoplasma gondii are the three main parasites found in transplant recipients.

- ***Cryptosporidium*** protozoa are spread via fecal-oral, animal-human, and waterborne routes. Cryptosporidium cause severe, persistent, watery diarrhea. Replace lost fluid; provide IV electrolytes, and nutritional support. Give IV spiramycin if dehydration develops.
- ***Strongyloides stercoralis*** is a parasitic worm that can live undetected for decades in the gastrointestinal tract, if the patient has strong immunity. However, after transplantation, disseminated strongyloidiasis can develop from immunosuppression. The larvae cause severe hemorrhagic enterocolitis and/or hemorrhagic pneumonia. Treatment is albendazole and ivermectin. If concomitant bacteremia or meningitis is present, provide systemic antibacterial therapy.
- ***Toxoplasma gondii*** cause toxoplasmosis, the third leading cause of food-borne death in the U.S. 60 million U.S. residents carry Toxoplasma from eating undercooked food, mother-to-child transmission, not washing fruit and vegetables, contaminated drinking water, handling cat litter, receiving contaminated blood, or working in a lab. Patients have flu symptoms, eye pain, seizures, nausea, and incoordination. Treatment is pyrimethamine, folinic acid, and sulfadiazine.

ORGANISMS AND DISEASES
HHV-6, HEPATITIS VIRUSES, POLYOMAVIRUS BK, AND POLYOMAVIRUS JC

The primary diseases caused by HHV-6, Hepatitis viruses, Polyomavirus BK, and Polyomavirus JC are discussed below:

- **HHV-6 (Human Herpes Virus 6):** This is NOT the type of virus that causes cold sores (herpes simplex 1) and genital herpes (herpes simplex 2). Instead, HHV-6 causes bone marrow suppression, encephalitis, and interstitial pneumonia. Symptoms include a rash, bone marrow dysfunction, malaise, and fever.

- **Hepatitis viruses:** Typically, the HBsAg test will be positive 2-6 months post-transplant. Symptoms can vary from mild gastrointestinal symptoms to sudden liver failure.
- **Polyomavirus BK:** Up to 60% of kidney transplant patients have latent BK, 5% develop obstructive nephropathy, and half of those with nephropathy lose their graft. BK causes tubulointerstitial nephritis and ureteral stenosis. Signs are fever, persistent hematuria, and elevated serum creatinine levels.
- **Polyomavirus JC:** JC infects the respiratory system, kidneys, or brain. JC causes multifocal demyelination and progressive neurological deficits. Up to 70% of the world's population may have a latent JC infection. Signs and symptoms of JC infection are: Vision loss; speech problems; loss of mental faculties; uncoordinated movements; paralysis; and coma.

RESPIRATORY SYNCYTIAL VIRUS, INFLUENZA VIRUS, AND VARICELLA ZOSTER

Respiratory syncytial virus (RSV) is a labile paramyxovirus that produces a characteristic fusion of human cells in tissue culture (the syncytial effect). RSV affects the entire respiratory system. Children are frequently carriers. RSV causes organ rejection through bronchiolitis obliterans. Symptoms of RSV include: Rhinorrhea; otalgia; cough; SOB; sinus congestion and sinusitis; and fever higher than 100.4°F.

Influenza virus (flu) can cause influenza syndrome for weeks and secondary bacterial complications. Signs and symptoms include: Fever; chills; unproductive cough; fatigue; headaches; sore throat; and myalgia. Young people are prone to cytokine storm from pandemic flu, with necrosis of fingers and toes.

Varicella zoster (chicken pox) can be localized skin vesicles or a disseminated infection. Localized dermatomal zoster involves two or three adjoining dermatomes without visceral involvement. Clinical manifestations of a disseminated infection include skin lesions, encephalitis, pancreatitis, hepatitis, and disseminated intravascular coagulation.

PARAINFLUENZA VIRUS, CORONAVIRUS, PARVOVIRUS B19, AND HUMAN PAPILLOMA VIRUS

Parainfluenza virus causes mild upper respiratory disease that may progress to pneumonia. Symptoms are usually mild and may imitate the flu.

Coronavirus causes severe acute respiratory syndrome (SARS). Signs and symptoms are: Fever above 100.4°F; headaches; cough; SOB; hypoxia; lymphopenia; thrombocytopenia; and mild increase in transaminases.

The only member of the **Parvoviridae** known to infect humans, **B19** causes: Refractory anemia; pancytopenia; thrombotic microangiopathy; fibrosing cholestatic hepatitis; and loss of graft function. Symptoms include: Chronic anemia; low platelets and WBC's; fever; malaise; and pancytopenia.

Human Papilloma Virus (HPV): Currently, there are over 100 different types of HPV identified. HPV causes: Cutaneous and genital warts; cervical and bladder cancer; squamous cell carcinoma; and anogenital carcinoma. Warts range from microscopic to large verrucas.

CENTRAL NERVOUS SYSTEMS SYNDROMES ASSOCIATED WITH TRANSPLANT RECIPIENTS

The four main central nervous systems syndromes associated with transplant recipients are:

- **Acute bacterial meningitis** from *Listeria monocytogenes* infection of the brain and spinal cord inflames the meninges and affects the cerebrospinal fluid surrounding the brain. Listeria in the soil, dust, or food enters the blood stream and migrates to the brain and spinal cord. Foods known to contain Listeria are lunchmeats, hot dogs, and soft cheese.
- **Chronic or subacute meningitis** has many associated pathogens, including: Cryptococcus neoformans; Mycobacterium tuberculosis; Coccidioides immitis; L. monocytogenes; Histoplasma capsulatum; Nocardia asteroides; and Strongyloides stercoralis.
- **Focal brain syndrome** is caused by Metastatic Aspergillus; L. monocytogenes; Toxoplasma gondii; and N. asteroides.
- **Progressive dementia** is caused by Polyomavirus JC; herpes simplex virus; cytomegalovirus; and Epstein-Barr virus).

LISTERIA MONOCYTOGENES, NOCARDIA, AND LEGIONELLA

Listeria monocytogenes causes: Nuchal rigidity; abdominal cramps; diarrhea; seizures; meningismus; focal neurological deficits; decreased level of consciousness (LOC); headaches; and a fever lasting 1-5 days. Preventative therapy for *Listeria monocytogenes* is to: Use only pasteurized dairy products and fruit juice; avoid soft cheeses; cook meats thoroughly; wash raw vegetables and fruits; keep your kitchen clean; and wash your hands frequently with soapy water.

Nocardia typically has a subacute onset. Symptoms include: Chest pain; cough; fever; pulmonary nodules; cavitating lesions; abscesses; infiltrates; and effusions. Patients may receive some protection against Pneumocystis pneumonia by taking prophylactic Trimethoprim/sulfamethoxazole (TMP-SMZ).

Legionella first manifests with flu-like symptoms (fever, chills, headaches, and malaise). It progresses to: Confusion; minimally productive cough; diarrhea; chest pain; and dyspnea. The best prevention for *Legionella* is to have Plant Operations and the Microbiology laboratory at the facility collect and test cultures from the hospital water supply and air filters routinely, and to use water treatments to manage nosocomial infections.

INFECTION ASSOCIATED WITH HEART ALLOGRAFT

The main types of infections associated with a **heart allograft** are:

- Ventilator-associated pneumonia
- Sternotomy infections

Ventilator-associated pneumonia is the result of Gram-negative bacteria such as *Pseudomonas, aeruginosa, Klebsiella pneumoniae*, and *Enterobacteriaceae*. A sternotomy infection is typically the result of coagulase-negative Staphylococci or *Staphylococcus aureus*. Other types of infections are mediastinitis (caused by Gram-negative bacteria), bacteremia, and bacterial pneumonia. Signs and symptoms that clinicians should look for include: Fever; leukocytosis; and systemic toxicity. Diagnosis of mediastinitis is usually via CT scan. Signs and symptoms of an *early* sternal wound infection include poor wound healing and dehiscence. *Late* signs and symptoms are sinus tract formation and purulent discharge. Treatment for both mediastinitis and a sternal wound infection is surgical wound debridement and antimicrobial therapy geared towards Gram-positive organisms.

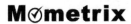

Pathogens Associated with Allograft Kidney Infections

80% of all **kidney infections** are bacterial. The entire urinary tract is involved if there is secondary bacteremia. Common pathogens linked to urinary tract infections are: *Enterobacteriaceae, Pseudomonas aeruginosa, and Enterococcus* sp. Risk factors associated with allograft kidney infections include: Diabetes; extended urinary catheter use; decreased urinary flow; neurogenic bladder; renal insufficiency; and anatomic abnormalities. Thwart allograft infections by removing the catheter early, and using TMP/SMX, cephalosporins, or Fluoroquinolones. Surgical wound infections can be treated preoperatively with cephalosporin antibiotics.

Infections of Pancreas Allografts Post-Transplantation

Common infections for **pancreas transplant** recipients include intra-abdominal abscesses, peritoneal infections with enteric bacteria, and urinary tract infections from indwelling catheters that lead to bacterial overgrowth in the bladder. Less common infections include abdominal wall cellulitis, peri-pancreatic abscesses, and peritonitis. Typically, Gram-positive cocci, Gram-negative bacteria, and anaerobic bacteria are to blame for these infections. Urinary tract infections are treated using a pathogen-specific antimicrobial such as Fluoroquinolones or Cephalosporin. Depending on the extent of the infection, wounds will most likely need surgical or scan guided drainage of the abscess. Preventative medications include TMP/SMX and Ciprofloxacin for urinary tract infections. If the patient has a sulfa allergy, Fluoroquinolones should be prescribed. Surgical wound infections can be prevented thought the use of perioperative cephalosporin.

Cholangitis and Roux-en-Y Choledochojejunostomy

Cholangitis is an infection of the biliary tract. Cholangitis has the potential to cause significant morbidity and mortality. **Roux-en-Y choledochojejunostomy** is a method used to repair the common bile duct. The most common sites of infection for a liver transplant recipient are the: Allograft; surgical site; biliary tract; peritoneal cavity; and bloodstream. Bacterial infections can occur through non-surgical wounds, cholangitis, abscesses, and device-related infections. Intra-abdominal infections can result from lengthy operations, CMV infection, blood transfusion, Roux-en-Y choledochojejunostomy, a re-operation, or re-transplantation. Signs and symptoms of infection include: Fever; abdominal pain; guarding; purulent drainage; and wound dehiscence. Diagnosis of a wound infection is made via cultures, a CT scan ultrasound, or MRI. Cholangitis is confirmed via a cholangiogram and liver function tests.

Non-Pharmacological Actions That Help Avoid Post-Transplant Infections

The recipient and his or her family should take these measures to **prevent infection**, especially during the first year post-transplant:

- Wash hands often with antimicrobial soap.
- Stay away from unpasteurized products.
- Wash raw fruits and vegetables thoroughly before eating.
- Avoid undercooked meats.
- Avoid animal sources of potential infections, such as litter boxes, feces and aquaria.
- Avoid contact with anyone who recently received a live virus vaccine, such as infants who are immunized for measles-mumps-rubella (MMR), varicella, and polio (with oral vaccine).
- Avoid all potential sources of fungal infections, like fresh flowers and live plants.
- Get an annual flu vaccine.
- Remove all indwelling lines and catheters as soon as the doctor deems it appropriate.
- Place a mask on the recipient patient when transporting him or her in the hospital.
- Use high-efficiency leukocyte blood filters.

Adhere to reverse isolation protocols.

NON-PHARMACOLOGIC INFECTION CONTROL MEASURES FOR PLANT OPERATIONS MANAGER AND OTHER HEALTHCARE STAFF

The **Plant Operations** manager at a transplant facility must:

- Monitor bathrooms, showers, and the air-condition system for Legionella.
- Use high-efficiency particulate air-filters (HEPA) in air-exchange systems

Healthcare staff must:

- Follow reverse isolation procedures.
- Limit visits into the patient's room by attending to all housekeeping and dietary needs.
- Use leukocyte-depleted, CMV-negative blood products for CMV-seronegative recipients.
- Use high-efficiency leukocyte blood filters.
- Disconnect all indwelling catheters as soon as possible.
- Acquire all post-transplant infection surveillance tests per protocol.

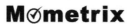

Post-Transplant Long-Term Complications

HYPOMAGNESEMIA

Hypomagnesemia is abnormally low levels of magnesium found in the blood. As a reference, use 1.8 to 2.5 mEq/L as the normal value. Hypomagnesemia occurs when the level is less than 1.8 mEq/L. The use of calcineurin inhibitors are correlated to low magnesium levels. The higher the blood concentration of calcineurin inhibitor levels, the lower the blood level of magnesium. Hypomagnesemia may be heightened in patients who are diabetic, pregnant, or taking diuretics. Clinical manifestations usually develop when the serum level falls below 1.0 mEq/L. The recommended regimen usually consists of magnesium replacement therapy. Be aware that over-the-counter magnesium supplements are costly and not always covered by insurance. Foods rich in magnesium include seafood, green vegetables, whole grains, and nuts.

GINGIVAL HYPERPLASIA

Gingival hyperplasia is an overgrowth of the gums as a common consequence of taking the immunosuppressant cyclosporin. Gingival hyperplasia worsens in patients who are excessive mouth breathers (adenoidal), or who have irritants such as plaque and calcified deposits on their teeth. The best way to minimize gingival hyperplasia is by routine dental scaling and checkups and, if possible, lowering the dose of cyclosporin. Another way to help reduce gingival hyperplasia is by using cyclosporin gel caps instead of liquid. In some patients, a possible substitute for cyclosporin is tacrolimus. If the condition becomes troublesome, oral surgery may be recommended.

GASTROINTESTINAL COMPLICATIONS FOLLOWING TRANSPLANTATION

Gastritis, peptic ulcers, perforated viscus, pancreatitis, and hepatitis are **common GI complications after organ transplantation**. Pancreatitis and hepatitis are both more difficult to diagnose in someone who has received a pancreas or liver transplant, respectively. Glucocorticoids therapy is habitually associated with GI irritation and hemorrhage. An antisecretory compound or H_2-histamine receptor antagonist is prescribed for 6-12 months after surgery, when steroid doses are highest. Even though most immunosuppressive medications are considered to play a major role in GI complications, the masking effects of these medications often avert or hinder identification of the problem. Hypercalcemia due to hyperparathyroidism can cause hemorrhaging after a renal transplant. Infections or superinfections with opportunistic organisms can end with inflammation and ulceration. Remember that mild and vague symptoms can lead to disastrous results if left untreated.

RENAL INSUFFICIENCY IN POST-TRANSPLANT RECIPIENTS

Immunosuppressive therapy is the primary cause of renal dysfunction; however, nephrotoxicity should be investigated in depth to rule out other causes. **Renal insufficiency** can be due to acute or chronic rejection, hypertension, diabetes, and dehydration. Reduce the calcineurin inhibitor dosage. Weigh the chance of kidney damage against the risk of precipitating rejection. It is more likely that nephrotoxicity will occur in the presence of high blood trough levels, but this is not always the case. Renal insufficiency can also occur in the presence of low blood trough levels. Other nephrotoxic medications include NSAIDS, diuretics, and antihypertensives.

HIGH CHOLESTEROL IN POST-TRANSPLANT PATIENTS

Pre-existing **hyperlipidemia** is most often the cause of post-transplant hyperlipidemia. Immunosuppressive agents are directly correlated to high serum lipid levels. Cyclosporin has been linked to elevated serum cholesterol and triglyceride levels. Tacrolimus, although linked to hyperlipidemia, is not as significant in the development of high cholesterol as cyclosporin is. Rapamycin has also been reported to raise cholesterol levels. To help combat hyperlipidemia, educate patients on the importance of healthy eating habits. If diet alone is not enough to lower serum lipid levels, initiate oral medications per order. The class of drugs called *statins* (3 hydroxy-3-methylglutaryl coenzyme A [HGM-CoA] reductase inhibitors) have been shown in studies to lower blood cholesterol in both the general population, and in solid organ transplant recipients. When taking statins, the patients risk developing rhabdomyolysis.

OSTEOPENIA AND OSTEOPOROSIS

Osteopenia is a reduction in bone volume, but not necessarily an increased risk of bone fractures. **Osteoporosis** is a loss of bone mass and density leading to bone fragility and an increased susceptibility to bone fractures. Hence, any degree of osteoporosis is a cause of concern. The World Health Organization (WHO) defines osteoporosis as a bone mineral density (BMD) greater than 2.5 standard deviations (SD) below the mean of young normal controls. Osteopenia is defined as bone mineral density (BMD) between 1 SD and 2.5 SD below young normal controls. Most transplant centers obtain a baseline bone density scan for all potential transplant recipients. Post-transplant bone density scans are compared with the baseline scan's findings. Most bone loss occurs during the first 6 months post-transplant; therefore, this is the most critical time to assess the patient for bone loss. 36% of transplant recipients experience a bone fracture(s) during the first year post-transplant.

> **Review Video: Osteoporosis**
> Visit mometrix.com/academy and enter code: 421205

SOLID ORGAN TRANSPLANT RECIPIENTS

Many times, there are pre-transplant factors that contribute to a solid organ recipient's chances of developing **osteoporosis**. Long-term complications that encourage development of osteoporosis include: Kidney failure; use of loop diuretics; prerenal azotemia; passive or active liver congestion; a history of smoking; hypogonadism; an inadequate intake of calcium; immunosuppressive therapy with steroids, cyclosporin (Neoral, Sandimmune, and Gengraf), Prograf, azathioprine, mycophenolate mofetil, and rapamycin. Of all of the drugs listed above, steroids are the most difficult immunosuppressive to manage because they are the building blocks of anti-rejection treatment in almost all types of solid organ transplants.

EFFECTS OF CORTICOSTEROID THERAPY ON BONE DENSITY

Corticosteroids affect bone density by the following methods:

- Increased calcium excreted by the kidneys.
- Reduced intestinal absorption of calcium.
- Increased parathyroid hormone levels.
- Decreased androgen levels.
- Decreased estrogen synthesis.
- Increased bone resorption.
- Decreased bone formation via osteoblasts.

Currently, the recommended dietary allowance (RDA) for all post-transplant recipients on steroid or calcineurin therapy is 1500 mg of calcium and 800-1000mg of vitamin D every day. If a patient has been diagnosed with osteoporosis and fractures by a DEXA scan, an inhibitor should be taken with the calcium and vitamin D. Examples of inhibitors are bisphosphonates (alendronate and etidronate), calcitonin, and estrogen. Bisphosphonates should be taken immediately in the morning with a full glass of water, 30 minutes before eating breakfast or drinking liquids. Sit upright for at least 30 minutes after taking biophosphates. Do not eat or drink for 30 minutes to allow for maximum absorption

POST-TRANSPLANT INSULIN THERAPY AND DIABETES

Many of the popular immunosuppressant medications on the market today are diabetogenic. Steroids have a great deal of influence on insulin resistance, glucose uptake, insulin receptor sensitivity, and insulin production. Studies show that cyclosporin and tacrolimus encourage insulin resistance, lower insulin secretion, and have a toxic effect on pancreatic beta cells. Treatment options for patients who develop diabetes post-transplant are very similar to the treatment plan for those with diabetes in the general population. Follow the Diabetes Control and Complications Trial (DCCT) guidelines. They recommend interventions for blood glucose levels over 126 mg/dl on two consecutive tests. Encourage the patient to keep his or her blood glucose level below 126 mg/dl to reduce the risk of end-organ damage.

POST-TRANSPLANT CANCER PREVENTION

Immunosuppressed organ recipients are at greater risk for developing **cancer**. Educate all transplant recipients and their families about cancer risks:

- Stop smoking and avoid second hand smoke.
- Perform routine skin examinations.
- Follow all routine cancer screening guidelines from the American Cancer Society:
    - See a dermatologist annually for a check-up and receive prompt treatment of any unusual findings.
    - Schedule a sigmoidoscopy or colonoscopy for all patients over 50.
    - Women should see their gynecologist annually for a Pap smear and mammogram, and perform monthly self breast examinations (SBE).
    - Men should have an annual prostate exam and a prostate-specific antigen test (PSA).
- Follow UV exposure precautions:
    - Do not use tanning beds.
    - Avoid unnecessary sun exposure.
    - Use sunscreen lotion with at least SPF 15.
    - Wear wide-brimmed hats, protective clothing, and sunglasses.

CANCER TREATMENT IN ORGAN TRANSPLANT RECIPIENT

On average, the incidence of cancer in solid organ transplant recipients is 6%. Transplant recipients have a tendency to develop cancer tumors that are considered to be unusual in the overall population. The key to successful treatment is early diagnosis. Follow all American Cancer Society screening recommendations. Lymphoma and post-transplant lymphoproliferative disease (PTLD) can be treated using Acyclovir and Ganciclovir, radiation therapy, or surgical excision of the infected lymph node. Decreasing immunosuppressive therapy can also be attempted. In some cases, all immunosuppressive therapies must be halted completely, and the patient must decide between the viability of the graft and life itself. Sadly, extrarenal transplant recipients have no alternative therapy to turn to if their grafts fail.

POST-TRANSPLANT SEXUAL DYSFUNCTION

For men, **impotence** is often present prior to transplantation, due to: Diabetes; coronary artery disease; high blood pressure; and beta-blockers used to treat congestive heart failure. If a man is not impotent prior to transplantation, often times he will develop impotence after a transplant, as a side-effect of immunosuppressive medications. **Sexual dysfunction and loss of libido** in women is typically related to the onset of menopause. Psychological factors also play an important role in female sexual dysfunction, including a fear of infection, fear of rejection, and a loss of intimacy.

CLINICIAN'S ROLE

Many patients never recover from sexual dysfunction post-transplant. The patient and his or her significant other may be too uncomfortable to discuss the problem or seek medical help. This is especially true when the health care provider is of the opposite sex. The clinical staff must take the initiative to gently introduce sexual dysfunction into the conversation, and put the patient and significant other at ease. Once such way to bring up the subject and validate its importance is to say, "Many people experience sexual problems following a transplant. Please discuss with me any changes you experience or concerns you may have." Depending on the cause of the sexual dysfunction, the patient may need to be referred to a urologist or gynecologist for further evaluation and treatment. Thanks to the widespread publicity for Viagra (sildenafil), the stigma once associated with sexual impotence has decreased.

Pharmacological Therapeutics

Immunosuppressives

IMMUNOSUPPRESSION, INDUCTION THERAPY, AND INITIAL IMMUNOSUPPRESSION

Immunosuppression is restraint of the immune system with drugs to encourage the body's acceptance of the allograft. Successful immunosuppression is preventing organ rejection while sustaining a satisfactory immune response against infections.

Induction therapy is a generic term for any immunosuppressive agent given prior to, or after, transplantation. Induction therapy is administered over a 1-2 week period. Two examples of induction therapy agents are monoclonal anti-CD3 antibodies (Muromonab-CD3) and polyclonal antilymphocyte antibodies (antilymphocyte globulin).

Initial immunosuppression indicates that an elevated dose of immunosuppressive therapy was administered immediately post-transplantation for graft maintenance.

IMMUNOSUPPRESSIVE AGENTS

The **protocol for immunosuppressive therapy** varies greatly among different transplant centers, depending on the type of organ transplant, patient population, and staff experience. As of this writing, the most widely-accepted immunosuppressive protocol is the combination of three separate medications: Calcineurin inhibitor; corticosteroid; and an antimetabolite agent. Factors that influence which immunosuppressive agents are prescribed include: Sex; race; age; procedure of each individual transplant center; and HLA incompatibility.

PROPER DOSAGE AND FACTORS THAT ALTER BLOOD LEVELS

Achieving proper immunosuppression is a delicate process. It requires finding the correct balance between effectiveness and safety. Overdosing or underdosing can cause organ rejection and toxic side effects. Currently, the best way to monitor for therapeutic levels is through blood analysis:

Drug	Monitoring Schedule
Cyclosporin	12-hour trough
Tacrolimus	12-hour trough
Mycophenolate mofetil	12-hour trough, WBC and platelet counts
Sirolimus	22-24 hour trough
Azathioprine	WBC and platelet counts

Factors that alter blood levels of immunosuppressive agents include: Multiple drug interactions; food reactions (e.g., grapefruit potentiates some medications, and milk slows absorption); variations in test type used by different labs to establish trough blood levels; noncompliance with medications; and pathophysiologic complications.

CALCINEURIN INHIBITORS

Calcineurin inhibitors: Calcineurin (CN) is a protein phosphatase responsible for triggering the transcription of interleukin, which encourages the growth and differentiation of the T-cell response.

Generic Name	Brand Name	Admin.
Cyclosporin USP	Sandimmune	oral, IV
Cyclosporin USP (modified)	Neoral	oral
Cyclosporin capsules USP (modified)	Gengraf	oral
Cyclosporin softgels USP	same	oral, IV
Tacrolimus, FK506	Prograf	oral
Sirolimus	Rapamune	oral

FOOD PRODUCTS TO AVOID

Calcineurin inhibitors (CNI) are commonly used to prevent allograft rejection. Studies have shown that taking calcineurin inhibitors in conjunction with **grapefruit** or **grapefruit juice** may alter the absorption effects of the medication. Initial studies of grapefruit taken with a calcineurin inhibitor were promising. However, no therapeutic dose of grapefruit could be established that would increase blood levels of the calcineurin inhibitor. Additional studies revealed variable and unpredictable increases in calcineurin drug levels with grapefruit consumption. *Warn patients that consuming grapefruit or grapefruit juice with a calcineurin inhibitor could result in drug toxicity.* Patients on calcineurin inhibitors should avoid grapefruit or grapefruit juice altogether, and substitute another citrus fruit, like orange juice.

MICROSOMAL ENZYMES

Condensed calcineurin inhibitor levels are affected by **microsomal enzymes**. There are two types of microsomal enzymes: P450 3A enzyme and Flavin mono-oxygenase (FMO3). In transplant cases, the enzyme most affected is P450 3A. When certain drugs inhibit P450 3A enzyme, the calcineurin inhibitor levels are augmented. Drugs that are inducers of cytochrome P450 3A can enhance drug metabolism, and cause a decline in calcineurin inhibitor levels.

ANTIMETABOLITES USED IN IMMUNOSUPPRESSIVE THERAPY

Antimetabolites*:* Agents that interfere with nucleotide syntheses and encourage anti-proliferation. Antimetabolites work by interrupting purine or pyrimidine biosynthesis on which T- and B-lymphocytes are selectively dependent.

Generic Name	Brand Name	Admin.
Azathioprine	Imuran	Oral, IV
Mycophenolate mofetil	CellCept	Oral, IV
Cyclophosphamide	Cytoxan	Oral, IV

IMMUNOSUPPRESSANTS PRESCRIBED AT COMPLETION OF INTESTINAL TRANSPLANT

Since 1990, the **principal immunosuppressant for post-intestinal transplant patients** has been tacrolimus (FK-506, Prograf, and Fujimycin). Thanks to tacrolimus, the survival rate of intestinal transplant recipients has increased considerably. Tacrolimus is usually administered in conjunction with a corticosteroid. During the intestinal transplant operation itself, tacrolimus is given continuously via an IV, at a rate of 0.15-0.2 mg/kg/day. Once GI motility returns, the route is switched to oral. The oral dose is usually 3-4 times the IV dose, divided into 2 doses daily. Blood levels of tacrolimus are usually sustained between 20 ng/ml-25ng/ml for 3 months. However, with

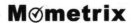

the occurrence of rejection, these levels may continue for up to 6 months. When patients are considered stable, blood levels should be decreased to 10-15 ng/ml by one year post-transplant.

IMMUNOSUPPRESSIVE PROTOCOL FOR POST-KIDNEY TRANSPLANT RECIPIENTS

Post operatively, **most kidney recipients will be on three separate therapies:** A corticosteroid; a calcineurin inhibitor; and Mycophenolate mofetil. Methylprednisolone remains the foundation block for most immunosuppression protocols. Usually, IV Methylprednisolone is given immediately post operatively, using the standard dose of 125 mg in a regimen of 6 separate doses. After that, the route switches from IV to oral Prednisone. The starting oral dose is typically 30 mg, which is tapered down to 20 mg, once it has been determined that the calcineurin inhibitor blood level is therapeutic. The preferred calcineurin inhibitor is tacrolimus or cyclosporin. If the patient has a history of calcineurin inhibitor toxicity, or if there are concerns about the length of the cold ischemia time, then the calcineurin inhibitor is held 3-5 days while induction therapy is given as an alternative. CellCept (Mycophenolate mofetil) is administered two times a day at 1-1.5 grams per dose. However, African Americans must be given a higher dose, due to an increased incidence of organ rejection.

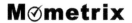

Non-Immunosuppressive Drugs

VANCOMYCIN HCL

The mechanism of action, indications, dosage, common side-effects and common drug interaction of Vancomycin are discussed below:

- *Mechanism of action:* Belongs to the family of glycopeptides; inhibits cell wall synthesis; bactericidal against Gram-positive bacteria with selective RNA synthesis.
- *Indications:* Vancomycin is used for prophylactic treatment of surgical infections in patients who are allergic to penicillin or Cephalosporin. Vancomycin may be taken when the probability of MRSA is high. It is used to treat staphylococcal species infections like staphylococcal endocarditis.
- *Dosage:* Adults with normal renal function: 2 g doses divided into 1 g every 12 hours for systemic infections. *Clostridium difficile* colitis is treated with 125 mg PO every 12 hours for 10-14 days. Pediatric patients with normal renal function: 10 mg/kg IV every 6 hours. The dose should run at least 60 minutes. (Note: This dosage may be lower in patients less than one month old.) Prophylaxis: 1 gm IV on call to the operating room
- *Common side effects:* Infusion reactions that are histamine-mediated, nephrotoxicity, neutropenia, and thrombocytopenia.
- *Common drug interactions:* Can decrease the effects of mycophenolate mofetil; increased risk of nephrotoxicity if taken with tacrolimus or cyclosporin.

METRONIDAZOLE (FLAGYL)

The mechanism of action, indications, dosage, common side-effects and common drug interactions of Flagyl are explained below:

- *Mechanism of action:* Cytotoxic to facultative anaerobic bacteria. Reductive action is by intracellular transport proteins. Metronidazole is reduced by pyruvate.
- *Indications:* A mainstay drug for the treatment of anaerobic infections; the treatment choice for diarrhea caused by *Clostridium difficile* colitis. FDA-approved for anaerobic and protozoal infections.
- *Dosage:* PO 250-500 mg TID or QID for 14 days (for the treatment of *C. diff*)
- *Common side effects:* Seek immediate medical attention for swelling of the face, tongue, throat, neck, or difficulty breathing. Other serious side effects include: Numbness or tingling in the hands or feet, pain or burning upon urinating and/or darkening of the urine, bloody or watery diarrhea, flu-like symptoms, including chills, sore throat, and body aches, metabolic taste disturbance, Leukopenia, Transient eosinophilia
- *Common drug interactions:* Tagamet increases blood levels of metronidazole. Flagyl should not be taken with amprenavir due to the presence of propylene glycol. Metronidazole may decrease the effect of mycophenolate mofetil because of a decrease in enterohepatic re-circulation. Tacrolimus and cyclosporin levels may be increased.

TRIMETHOPRIM/SULFAMETHOXAZOLE

The mechanism of action, indications, dosage, common side-effects and common drug interactions of Trimethoprim/sulfamethoxazole are discussed below:

- *Mechanism of action:* An antibacterial combination drug with two different agents that act in succession to prevent the biosynthesis of nucleic acids.
- *Indications:* Prescribed for urinary tract infections, inflammation of the intestines, middle ear infections, bronchitis, *Pneumocystis Carinii*, pneumonitis, *Toxoplasma gondii, Nocardia sp.*, and *Listeria monocytogenes.*
- *Dosage:* Post-transplant 80/400 or 160/800 PO QD to 3 X week for 3-12 months
- *Common side effects:* Transient eosinophilia, leukopenia, n/v, loose stools, dyspepsia, and metabolic taste disturbance.
- *Common drug interactions:* Can increase Voriconazole levels because sulfamethoxazole is a CYP P450 2C9 inhibitor; can decrease the effect of mycophenolate mofetil because of a drop in enterohepatic re-circulation.

CEFAZOLIN SODIUM

The mechanism of action, indications, dosage, common side-effects and common drug interactions of Cefazolin Sodium are explained below:

- *Mechanism of action:* Bactericidal; first-generation Cephalosporin; interferes with cell wall synthesis.
- *Indications:* Prophylactic treatment of surgical site infections. Can treat Gram-negative and Gram-positive organisms, including methicillin-susceptible *Staph aureus*, PCN-susceptible *Strep pneumoniae,* Group B *Streptococc*i, and *S. viridans*.
- *Dosage:* Prophylactic treatment on call to OR: 1 gm IV. Treatment of tissue infections: 1 gm IV Q8h.
- *Common Side Effects:* Flu-like symptoms; joint pain; rash; urticaria; diarrhea; colitis; and headaches.
- *Common Drug Interactions:* Can cause a decrease in enterohepatic recirculation, which may decrease the efficacy of mycophenolate.

ACYCLOVIR

Acyclovir is a nucleoside analog, which selectively inhibits the replication of herpes simplex virus (Types 1 and 2). After the intracellular uptake has occurred, Acyclovir is converted to acyclovir triphosphate. Acyclovir triphosphate selectively inhibits DNA synthesis and viral replication. Acyclovir is active in vitro against both HSV Types 1 and 2, *Varicella zoster*, Epstein-Barr virus, *herpesvirus simiae*, and cytomegalovirus. Acyclovir is used in the treatment and suppression of shingles, chickenpox and HSV. Dosage strength depends on the indications, as follows:

- Herpes zoster: 800 mg PO 5x/day x 7-10 days
- Chickenpox: 800 mg PO 4-5x/day x 5-7 days
- HSV: 200 mg PO 5x/day x 10 days OR 400 mg PO TID x 7-10 days
- Chronic suppressive therapy: 400 mg PO BID x 12 months (maximum)
- IV dosage: 5-20 mg/kg IV q 8h x 5-10 days

Renal function must be considered and dosage adjustments made accordingly. Common side-effects include nephrotoxicity, an increase in liver enzymes, headaches, and GI symptoms.

VALACYCLOVIR

Valacyclovir (Valtrex) is a prodrug that is converted by the hepatic first pass metabolism by esterases to an active drug named acyclovir. Acyclovir is then converted to monophosphate (this monophosphate state plays a critical role in the halting of DNA replication, resulting in chain termination). The monophosphate form is further broken down into an active triphosphate form known as acyclo-GTP. Acyclo-GTP is an extremely strong inhibitor of viral DNA polymerase (an enzyme that assists in DNA replication). Indications for Valtrex are the treatment and suppression of cold sores (herpes labialis), shingles (herpes zoster), and genital herpes. The dosage of Valacyclovir depends on the indication, as follows:

- Cold sores: 2000 mg PO q 12 hours x 2 doses
- Shingles: 1,000 mg PO TID x 7 days
- Genital herpes: 1000 mg PO BID x 7-10 days for the first episode; 500 mg BID x 3-5 days for all recurrent episodes

Renal function must be considered and dosage adjustments made accordingly. Common side-effects include nephrotoxicity, an increase in liver enzymes, headaches, and GI symptoms.

GANCICLOVIR

The primary action of **Ganciclovir** (also known as Cytovene or Cymevene), is to inhibit the replication of viral DNA through ganciclovir-5'-triphosphate. Ganciclovir is metabolized to the triphosphate mainly through 3 nucleotide-metabolizing enzymes: deoxyguanosine kinase, guanylate kinase, and phosphoglycerate kinase. The indication for Ganciclovir is to prevent and treat cytomegalovirus disease. The dosage for Ganciclovir depends on the indication, as follows:

- Induction: 5 mg/kg x 14-21 days IV; each dose to infuse over 1 hour
- Maintenance: 5 mg/kg IV x 7 days/week OR 6 mg/kg q day x 5 days/week OR 1000 mg PO TID
- CMV retinitis induction: 5 mg/kg 12 hours x 14-21 days IV
- CMV retinitis maintenance: 5 mg/kg x 7 days IV OR 1,000 mg PO TID
- CMV prevention: 1,000 mg PO TID

Each IV dose is to infuse over one hour. Oral dose must be administered with food. Renal function must be considered and dosage adjustments made accordingly. Side- effects include nephrotoxicity, increased liver enzymes, neurotoxicity, hematological toxicity, GI upset, fever, chills, phlebitis, and pruritus.

VALGANCICLOVIR

Valganciclovir (Valcyte) is the L-valyl ester of Ganciclovir. Valganciclovir is swiftly and extensively converted to Ganciclovir upon entering the human body. The advantage of oral Valganciclovir over Ganciclovir is its ability to attain *in vitro* exposure similar to IV Ganciclovir and higher than oral Ganciclovir doses. The indication for Valganciclovir is to treat CMV retinitis in AIDS patients. The dosage for Valganciclovir depends on the indication, as follows:

- Induction: 900 mg PO BID x 21 days
- Maintenance: 900 mg PO QD
- CMV prevention: 900 mg PO QD

Oral Valganciclovir must be administered with food. Renal function must be considered and dosage adjustments made accordingly. Common side-effects of Valganciclovir are very similar to

Ganciclovir's, and include nephrotoxicity, increased liver enzymes, neurotoxicity, hematological toxicity, GI upset, fever, chills, phlebitis, and pruritus.

FAMCICLOVIR

Upon intracellular uptake, **Famciclovir** (Famvir) is quickly converted to Penciclovir. Penciclovir triphosphate, in the active form, hinders DNA polymerase competitively with deoxyguanosine triphosphate and is incorporated into the extending DNA. Famciclovir is used in the treatment and suppression of cold sores (herpes labialis), shingles (herpes zoster), and genital herpes. The dosage for Famciclovir depends on the indication, as follows:

- Genital herpes: 250 mg PO TID x 7-10 days for first episode; 125 mg BID x 5 days for all recurrent episodes
- Cold sores: 125-150 mg PO BID x 5 days
- Shingles: 500 mg PO TID x 7 days

Renal function must be considered and dosage adjustments made accordingly. Common side-effects of Famciclovir include fatigue, GI upset, pruritus, headaches and dizziness.

LAMIVUDINE

Lamivudine (Epivir) is a synthetic nucleoside (dideoxynucleoside analogue) which has activity against HIV-1 and HBV. The chief mode of action of Lamivudine is the inhibition of HIV-1 reverse transcriptase via DNA chain termination. Lamivudine is the first nucleoside analogue approved to treat chronic HBV infections. Lamivudine is primarily used in the treatment of patients with diagnosed or suspected hepatitis B. The dosage for Lamivudine is 100 mg PO QD with adjustments made for renal function. Side-effects include fatigue and malaise, respiratory infections, and GI symptoms such as nausea, vomiting, abdominal discomfort and pain, and diarrhea.

FLUCONAZOLE

Fluconazole is a broad-spectrum antifungal. Fluconazole inhibits ergosterol synthesis in the cell wall of yeast and fungi. It is a highly selective inhibitor of fungal cytochrome P450 sterol C-14 alpha-demethylation in the cell membrane. Fluconazole is used in the treatment of candidiasis and cryptococcal meningitis. The dosage depends on the location of the candidiasis. *Fluconazole is not recommended for children under the age of 6 months.*

- Vulvovaginal candidiasis: 150 mg PO x 1 dose
- Oropharyngeal candidiasis: 200 mg PO x 1 dose followed by 100 mg PO daily x 2 weeks
- Tinea pedis, cruris, corporis: 50 mg PO daily x 2-6 days

Renal function must be considered and dosage adjustments made accordingly. Common side-effects of Fluconazole include an increase in liver enzymes, stomach upset, headaches, and rash.

ITRACONAZOLE

The mechanism of action for **Itraconazole** is basically the same as all other azole antifungals—the synthesis of P450 oxidase-mediated synthesis of ergosterol is inhibited.

Itraconazole is an antifungal that has a broader spectrum of activity than Fluconazole does. However, Itraconazole is not as broad as Voriconazole. Itraconazole is effective against invasive and non-invasive aspergillosis, whereas Fluconazole is not. It is also effective against candidiasis, histoplasmosis, sporotrichosis, para-coccidioidomycosis, chromomycosis, blastomycosis, dermatomycosis, and onychomycosis. Itraconazole has almost zero penetration into the cerebrospinal fluid and is almost 99% protein bound. Itraconazole is available in oral solution, capsules, and IV form. The standard dose is 100 to 400 mg PO daily or 200 mg IV daily. Renal function must be considered and dosage adjustments made accordingly. Side-effects include elevated alanine aminotransferase levels, increased toxicity to CYP P430 3A4 metabolized medications, and a decreased efficacy of Itraconazole.

VORICONAZOLE

Voriconazole (Vfend) is a triazole antifungal agent that is a highly selective inhibitor of the cytochrome P450 sterol C-14-alpha-lanosterol demethylation located in the fungi's cell membrane. The P450 sterol C-14-alpha-lanosterol demethylation is a crucial step in fungal ergosterol biosynthesis. Voriconazole is used in the treatment of deadly fungal infections such as invasive aspergillosis. The dosage of Voriconazole is as follows:

- IV loading dose: 6 mg/kg x 2 doses 12 hours apart
- Maintenance dose: 4 mg/kg Q 12 hours
- Oral loading dose: 400 mg Q 12 hours x 2 doses
- Oral maintenance dose: 200mg Q day

If the patient weighs less than 20 kg, give 100 mg Q day. Renal function must be considered and dosage adjustments made accordingly. Side-effects include hepatoxicity, vision changes, GI upset, headaches, fever, and rash.

CLOTRIMAZOLE

Clotrimazole is an azole broad-spectrum antifungal agent that damages the fungal cell wall and, as a result, alters its permeability. It also inhibits the activity of the intracellular enzyme 2, 4-methylenedihydrol-anosterol to demethylsterol. Demethylsterol is the precursor to ergosterol. Ergosterol is a vital building block of the cytoplasmic membrane of the fungi. Clotrimazole is used prophylactically and in the treatment for oropharyngeal candidiasis. The dosage is as follows:

- Prophylaxis: 10 mg PO TID x 3-6 months
- Treatment: 10 mg PO 5 x day for 14 days

Patients should be advised to suck on troches and not chew or swallow them whole. Side-effects include visual changes, fever, rash, abdominal pain, nausea/vomiting, diarrhea, headaches, sepsis, peripheral edema, and rash.

TREATING POST-TRANSPLANT RECIPIENTS WITH HIGH BLOOD PRESSURE

Hypertension in post-transplant recipients must be treated immediately and aggressively. Educate patients who develop hypertension and encourage them to incorporate positive health behaviors into their routine schedules. Examples of positive health behaviors include: Weight loss, if necessary; implementing an exercise routine; smoking cessation, if applicable. These interventions alone will most likely not be enough to control high blood pressure that is brought on by a calcineurin-inhibitor. A calcium channel blocker may be prescribed in order to attain blood pressure control. If health-promoting activities are combined with a calcium channel blocker, it is possible that the patient will need a lesser dose of medication, because they have a synergistic effect. Current data suggests that tacrolimus induces less hypertension than cyclosporin. Therefore, it is of high importance to tailor the immunosuppressive therapy to each individual patient.

Education and Discharge

Discharge Education

EFFECTS OF RELIGIOUS BELIEFS AND ETHNICITY ON PROCESS OF LEARNING

In some situations, clinicians find themselves dealing with over-protective families. The family may wish that the nurse provides education directly to them, but bypass the patient. It is important to understand that the patient's family does this as a way to spare the patient from stressful information or bad news. In other situations, the family may request that all teaching be deferred until the patient's health has improved. Clinicians may find it beneficial to conduct teaching separately in these circumstances. The family needs to understand that, in order for the patient to make an informed decision regarding transplantation, he or she must know the risks and benefits involved. Certain cultural practices limit or prevent teaching session during certain times of the day and on certain days. Judaism prohibits teaching on the Sabbath. Jehovah's Witnesses will decline a blood transfusion.

IDENTIFYING WHEN PATIENT IS PREPARED TO BE TAUGHT

In order to be **ready to received education**, the patient must first accept his or her diagnosis, before instructions can be retained. Once diagnosis acceptance is well established and the initial anger has passed, then the patient is ripe for teaching. If the patient is in denial about the diagnosis, he or she may believe spontaneous recovery will occur, and a transplant can be avoided. If denial presents itself, provide the patient with age-appropriate educational material. For adults and older teens, include outcome data on the appropriate type of end-stage disease. Prior to beginning an educational session, assess the patient's physical and mental health status. Postpone the educational session if the patient is fragile or in extreme pain. Obtain a translator, if necessary.

FOUR STAGES OF LEARNING

The *Four Stages of Learning* is Susan Setley's theory that complete learning is processed in four stages: Exposure, guided learning, independence, and mastery. Setley's theory is particularly appropriate for transplant recipients.

1. **Exposure:** Present new concepts or ideas, starting when the patient and family initially meets with transplant coordinators. Do not overwhelm them with great detail.
2. **Guided learning:** Teach the patient about self-care. Teach the patient and family about complex medications and long-term care. Increase the level of detail.
3. **Independence:** Prior to discharge, help the patient and family to gain self-sufficiency through answering their questions, rehearsing what they have already learned, and repeating back the key elements. Use positive reinforcements.
4. **Mastery:** During this final step, observe the patient and family to ensure they have accomplished the goal, and are capable of successful long-term self-care. Congratulate them and provide a list of contact numbers.

EXPOSURE PHASE

The **exposure phase** of the Four Stages of Learning occurs at the initial meeting between the patient, his or her family, and transplant staff. It is during this first stage that the learning process begins. Invest great effort into this initial meeting, because it will set the attitude for all meetings to come. The nurse must address many complex issues with the family. Explain the:

- Evaluation process for becoming a potential organ donor.
- Waiting list for a new organ.
- Organ distribution system.
- Describe the surgery, and make it specific to that individual.
- Time the patient can expect to remain in the hospital post-transplant.
- Complications to expect after surgery.
- Evaluation process, which will include lab work, referring physicians, and tests.
- Follow-up care and doctor visits.
- Post-transplantation quality of life.
- Specific organ transplantation summary.

ACTIVITY GUIDELINES FOR LIVING LIVER DONORS FOLLOWING DISCHARGE FROM HOSPITAL

After **discharge**, educate all donors to start a program of daily exercise. The schedule should include aerobic exercises such as walking or using a stationary bike. The purpose is to gradually build strength and endurance. Advise the patients to make gradual, incremental increases over a period of about two months. Instruct patients not to lift, push, or pull anything over 15 pounds during their recovery time. Explain to the patients why they must report any adverse reactions immediately, and give them a list of pertinent phone numbers. Often, donors need a great deal of encouragement to pursue their exercise regimens, because they experience severe fatigue. They may fear harming their livers, or dread pain and discomfort. Closely monitor the donors' emotional states.

EDUCATIONAL CURRICULUM FOR SOLID ORGAN TRANSPLANT RECIPIENT

Create a **curriculum** that involves all senses, rather than a single-facet approach. Learners are kinesthetic, auditory, or visual. Accordingly, the more senses an educator is able to include in a teaching session, the greater the chance that all different types of learners will retain the material taught. Encourage interaction from the patient through note-taking, question-and-answer session, hands-on demonstrations, and give anecdotal examples of all important concepts to be retained. Listening to material in lecture format will engage auditory learners, but retention is poor. Use posters or a PowerPoint slide presentation to involve the visual learners. Note-taking provides tactile stimulation for kinesthetic learners. Finally, request that both the patient and family return to demonstrate all information taught, as reinforcement.

EDUCATIONAL MATERIAL FOR REGAINING AUTONOMY

Prior to discharge, present educational material in much more depth than the material covered prior to transplantation. Post-transplant patients begin to participate in their own care with backing and supervision from the clinical staff. Prior to discharge from the hospital, the patient needs to be able to demonstrate some independence. Adults and teenagers must be able to self-medicate. They must be able to: Identify each drug; state what it is used for; understand its side effects; know the correct dosage, route, and schedule. Patients must be able to describe with accurate detail the signs and symptoms of infection and organ rejection. Give patients handouts of slide shows previously used as audiovisual material. PowerPoint handouts provide instant summaries of the most important information.

Transplant Precautions

PRECAUTIONS FOR USING WELL WATER

Chlorinated tap water and bottled water are considered safe to drink without the need for boiling, chemical treatment, or additional filtration. However, **transplant recipients must always boil well water first, before consuming it or bathing in it.** Well water carries these infectious organisms that could be fatal if used by someone in an immunosuppressed state: *E-coli O157:H7; Giardia lamblia; Legionella pneumophila;* and other gram-negative organisms. Untreated well water used for showering causes these organisms to become airborne, where they can infect by ingestion, inhalation, or contact. Nausea, diarrhea, and fever can take a week to develop. In May 2000, *E-coli* killed six people, sickened 700, and caused mass kidney damage in Walkerton, when the town's water supply was contaminated with cattle manure from farm run-off after a storm. Educate all transplant patients about well water safety. Water can be tested by contacting the local water company, or by calling the EPA Safe Water Hotline at (800) 426-4791.

AVOIDANCE OF PETS

Most **pets** are considered safe and acceptable for recipients after transplantation, because pets promote the recovery process by enhancing emotional and psychosocial well-being. **Transplant patients must avoid**: Baby chicks and ducklings; turtles, lizards, and snakes; monkeys; farm animals; animals under 6 months old; ill or stray animals. Never recommend that an *already existing* pet be separated from the transplant recipient. If the patient does not have a pet at the time of the transplant, express the need to *wait at least one year* before getting one. Birds and reptiles carry *Salmonella, Chlamydia psittaci,* and *Cryptococcus.* Transplant recipients should not clean aquariums or bird cages. Pet dogs must be immunized against *Bordetella bronchiseptica* (kennel cough) if they will be around a lung transplant patient, and the transplant recipient must not clean up dog stools. Tell the transplant recipient to let another household member clean the cat's litter box daily, because it can transmit toxoplasmosis.

RECOMMENDATIONS FOR PET OWNERS

The following are educational recommendations that should be given to transplant recipients who are pet owners:

- Avoid cleaning body fluids from sick pets; if you must, wear disposable gloves.
- Designate a responsible, healthy adult to provide daily care for pets during the first year after transplant.
- Feed pet commercial food; if you give human food as a treat, cook it well or make sure it is pasteurized.
- Do not allow pet to drink from the toilet, eat other animals' droppings, hunt, or scavenge garbage.
- If pets get sick, confine and consult a vet.
- If you must change the litter box, wear a mask and gloves because cats can carry toxoplasmosis, a parasite that causes blindness and brain damage.
- Treat scratches immediately, before they become infected.
- Keep pets inside, except dogs on supervised walks.
- Do not sleep with your pets.
- Avoid other people's pets.
- Wash your hands with warm, soapy water after each time you handle a pet, clean its cage, or change its litter.

STRATEGIES FOR PATIENTS TO UNDERSTAND THE MEDICATION SYSTEM

Transplant medications are complex and difficult to understand for the lay person. Devise **simple reminders to decrease confusion**, for example:

- Usually a standard pillbox is not large enough to accommodate all of the medications a transplant recipient must take in a week. An easy solution is a tackle box. Ask the patient to purchase a fishing tackle box or craft box with compartments. Each column can represent a day of the week, and each row can represent the time of day. Label the columns accordingly (morning, evening, mid-afternoon, night).
- Have the patient purchase small and large zip-lock bags. The small bags represent specific doses to be taken throughout the day. The larger bags represent the days of the week. Be sure to label all bags accordingly.

Remember that each patient is different, and what works for one patient may not work for the next. For that reason, it is important to always individualize the medication system.

HELPING PATIENT BE COMPLIANT WITH PRE-AND-POST-TRANSPLANT REGIMENS

Most patients and their families find medical regimens to be very complicated and overwhelming. **Help patients to be compliant** and responsible for their own care by using these methods:

- Teach the patient how to keep a journal to record weights, vital signs, changes in medications, medical appointments, and any questions for the transplant team. Review the journal at every appointment, and answer any questions.
- Enroll the patient and family in a pharmacy program that is transplant-specific. Transplant-specific programs help simplify the medication-ordering process.
- Use every single opportunity with the patient as a time for teaching. Ask the patient to review important information.
- Assist the patient and family to develop an easy-to-understand medication schedule

Professional Responsibilities

Transplantation Research

KEY RESOURCES OF TRANSPLANTATION RESEARCH

Key **resources** for transplantation research that a nurse can utilize to stay up-to-date in best practices include:

- **Journals**: Journal of Heart and Lung Transplantation, American Journal of Transplantation, Clinical Journal of the American Society of Nephrology, Bone Marrow Transplantation, Liver Transplantation, Transplant International, Transplantation, Transplantation Research, Pediatric Transplantation, American Nurse Today, American Journal of Nursing, Journal of Research in Nursing, Journal of Evidence-Based Medicine, International Journal of Evidence-Based Healthcare.
- **Databases**: SRTR database, Cochrane Library, PubMed, CINAHL Plus, and Excerpt Medica Database (EMBASE).
- **Professional organizations**: International Transplant Nurses Society, Organization for Transplant Professionals (NATCO), American Organ Transplant Association, American Society of Transplantation.
- **Books**: Textbook of Organ Transplantation (Kirk, Knechtle and Larsen, 2014), Atlas of Organ Transplantation (Humar and Sturdevant, 2015), Contemporary Liver Transplantation (Doria, 2017), Organ Transplantation in Times of Donor Shortage (Jox, Assadi, and Marckmann, Eds, 2016).

NURSE'S ROLE IN CONTRIBUTING TO TRANSPLANTATION RESEARCH AND EDUCATION

The nurse's role in contributing to **transplantation research and education** includes:

- Serving as an advocate to ensure that the patient's rights are respected and that the patient has made informed consent regarding research.
- Carrying out literature research on topics of interest.
- Keeping current in information through continuing education and other courses.
- Identifying areas of interest for research.
- Applying for grants to fund research.
- Documenting carefully all patient care.
- Identifying potential test subjects and enrolling subjects when appropriate.
- Utilizing effective communication skills with team members and supporting organizations.
- Giving presentations to the bioethics committee, board of directors, and administrators regarding research proposals.
- Collecting, collating, and assessing data.
- Collecting specimens at point of care (blood, urine, stool, discharge).
- Ensuring that the protocol for research is implemented correctly.
- Educating peers about research.
- Writing reports, journal articles, and educational handouts.
- Participating in professional organizations.

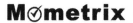

Legal/Ethical Issues

ETHICAL PRINCIPLES RELEVANT TO LIVING ORGAN DONATIONS

Autonomy is self-determination. The decision to commit to surgery resides with the donor. In order to make an autonomous decision, the donor must be able to comprehend the potential benefits and dangers of an organ transplant. Donors must be free from any external pressure that could influence their decision.

Beneficence is putting the patient's safety and interests above all else. Beneficence may require the medical and surgical staff to withhold requested treatment options that will cause more damage than good.

Nonmaleficence is the Hippocratic Oath: "First, do no harm." Doctors must make certain that the measures they offer to patients will provide the most benefit with the least potential amount of damage.

Justice means treating all patients impartially. The distribution of limited transplant organs is performed without regard to financial gain, celebrity status, or other prejudices.

ROLE OF BIOETHICS IN ORGAN TRANSPLANTATION

Organ transplantation is a **bioethical issue** that falls under the purview of the bioethics committee. The primary goal of bioethics committee is to determine the most morally correct action using the set of circumstances given. Bioethics committees are usually comprised of a number of diverse individuals, including physicians, nurses, community members, administrators, educators, attorneys, and spiritual advisors. Members are responsible for understanding issues related to bioethics and ethical analysis. Bioethics committees establish policies and procedures related to ethical concerns, provide consultation to help to resolve ethical problems or dilemmas, and educate others about ethical issues. The primary concerns of bioethics committees are that the rights of patients be respected and that patients and caregivers arrive at decisions through a process of sharing. If the patients/families and the healthcare providers agree when it comes to values and decision-making, then no ethical dilemma exists; however, when there is a difference in value beliefs, there is a bioethical dilemma that must be resolved. Sometimes, discussion and explanation can resolve differences, but at times the institution's bioethics committee must be brought in to resolve the conflict.

ETHICAL DILEMMAS IN ORGAN TRANSPLANTATION

Common **ethical dilemmas** that present themselves in organ transplantation include:

- **Selection of candidates/recipients:** Determining who receives an organ can pose a dilemma pitting the old against the young, unhealthy against unhealthier. Centers typically limit transplantations in those over a certain age. Another dilemma occurs regarding who "deserves" a transplant—someone who needs an organ through no fault or someone who, for example, needs an organ because of substance abuse.
- **Harvesting before brain death (anencephaly):** Some authorities believe that organs from infants with anencephaly should be harvested prior to technical brain death while others believe that the infant should be first declared brain dead.
- **Organ trafficking:** Organs are obtained through fraud, coercion, or abuse of power and given to those who can afford to pay exorbitant costs. In some cases, people willingly sell their organs, such as a kidney are part of a liver. This most often occurs outside of the United States with the poor being victimized by the wealthy.

LEGAL FRAMEWORKS IN ORGAN TRANSPLANTATION REGARDING DECLARATION OF BRAIN DEATH

The Uniform Determination of Brain Death Act requires that **brain death** be determined by accepted medical standards and findings of irreversible loss of all brain function although the heart may continue to beat. The ventilator must be discontinued and the patient declared dead before organ donation. Indications of brain death include:

- **Coma**: The cause of irreversible coma should be determined, excluding recent use of drugs that depress CNS, hypothermia, or neuromuscular blocking agents. Severe acid-base, endocrine, or electrolyte imbalances should be absent. The patient should not exhibit motor response or eye movement to stimuli and testing of brainstem reflexes (pupillary, ocular movement, corneal, facial muscle, pharyngeal, tracheal) should show absence.
- **Apnea**: Apnea testing involving removing the patient from the ventilator should be carried out. Confirmatory testing may also be done, especially if apnea testing is indeterminate.
- **Absence of brain stem reflexes**: Testing of brainstem reflexes:
  - Pupillary, ocular movement, and cornea: Bilateral response to light, oculocephalic and oculovestibular testing with observation for one minute.
  - Facial muscle: Response to stimuli.
  - Pharyngeal, tracheal: Tongue blade and/or suction catheter used to test gag reflex and cough response.

APNEA TEST TO DETERMINE BRAIN DEATH

The **apnea test** is an important element in the determination of brain death. Hypotension (at least 90 mm Hg), hypovolemia, and hypoxia must be corrected and normothermia (36.5° C/97° F) and eucapnia ($PaCO_2$ 35 to 45 mm Hg) achieved in order to obtain an accurate assessment:

- Preoxygenate for 30 minutes (100%).
- Obtain ABGs if oxygen saturation is not 95% or above.
- Disconnect ventilator but administer oxygen through ETT (100% at 8L/min) or nasal cannula (to carina level) to ensure oxygenation and observe for respiratory movement.
- Stop procedure and reconnect ventilator if systolic BP falls below 90 mm Hg and/or oxygen saturation falls to 85% for 30 seconds or arrhythmias occur and repeat ABGs.
- Otherwise, with no signs of respirations, repeat ABGs in 10 minutes and reconnect the ventilator.
- If PCO_2 is 60 mm Hg or >20 mm Hg over baseline normal the apnea test supports brain death.
- If PCO_2 is <60 mm Hg or increase is <20 mm Hg over baseline normal, test is indeterminate and confirming tests are required. Various confirming tests may be carried out: EEG, ultrasound, cerebral scintigraphy, cerebral angiography.

LEGAL FRAMEWORKS IN ORGAN TRANSPLANTATION REGARDING DECLARATION OF CIRCULATORY DEATH

Circulatory death (AKA cardiac death) involves irreversible loss of function of the heart and lungs. Organ donation after circulatory determination of death (DCDD) is possible only with controlled DCDD in which CPR will not be attempted and loss of circulation is permanent and not after unsuccessful CPR has been performed and loss of circulation is irreversible. However, donations can occur after uncontrolled loss of circulation with an unplanned cardiac arrest in a patient with a DNR. The patient must be declared dead (Dead donor rule), verified by tests/procedures, before donation, and the decision to forego CPR by the patient or family must have been separate from decisions about organ donation. The patient is extubated and typically observed for 5 minutes of mechanical asystole to ensure that spontaneous resuscitation of pulmonary or cardiac function does not occur prior to a declaration of death. Tests that may be used to validate circulatory absence include ultrasound, echocardiogram, and intra-arterial pulse monitoring.

LEGAL FRAMEWORKS REGARDING LIVING DONORS

Living donors are those who donate an organ (kidney) or part of an organ (liver) to another individual. Living donations may be directed at a specific person (usually a relative), non-directed (to an unknown recipient), or paired (two pairs of donors and recipients who do not match trade with each other to provide a matching donor for each recipient). The donor must freely make the organ donation and must have a clear understanding of medical/psychological risks (pain, infection, bile leakage, reduced kidney function in remaining kidney, hernia, intestinal perforation, hemorrhage). The donor must undergo medical, ethical, and psychosocial assessments to ensure readiness for donation. The donor must consider insurance coverage in the event complications occur and are not covered as well as the costs of taking time off from work for up to 8 weeks. The donor must not have been coerced into donation, must make informed consent, and must agree to donation willingly without expecting personal gain (including monetary payments).

NEW TRENDS IN ORGAN DONATION/TRANSPLANTATION

New trends in organ donation/transplantation include:

- Increased focus on organ donation after circulatory determination of death (DCDD).
- Increased paired donations.
- Expansion of organ donation to include more other organs or body parts, such as the penis, uterus, and face.
- Increased focus on regenerative medication and use of stem cells to make synthetic implants, such as tracheas.
- Increased numbers of living donors for both directed and non-directed transplantation.
- Further discussion regarding the ethics of organ donations.
- Increased need for organ donation, including longer wait list and wait time.
- Better immunosuppressive/antirejection regimens.
- Increased numbers of deceased donors, including from ethnic minorities.
- Improved methods of preserving organs for transplantation.
- Expanded criteria for recipients, such as accepting recipients at an older age.
- Increased reliance on foreign patients who pay cash for transplantation to offset costs.
- Increased donations from donors who die of overdose.
- Increased research regarding donation/transplantation.

CCTN Practice Test

1. The metabolic abnormality associated with end-stage liver disease and uremia is

    a. metabolic acidosis.
    b. metabolic alkalosis.
    c. respiratory acidosis.
    d. respiratory alkalosis.

2. The type of insulin most commonly used to treat hyperglycemia post-cardiac transplantation is

    a. intermediate-acting NPH insulin, Humulin N, or Novolin N.
    b. short-acting regular insulin, such as Novolin R.
    c. long-acting (glargine) Lantus insulin.
    d. rapid-acting (lispro H) Humalog or (aspart) NovoLog.

3. Prior to transplantation, a patient must undergo transplant-specific lab work. Which of the following screening tests are routinely performed pre-transplantation?

    I. ABO blood typing, human leukocyte antigen (HLA), and panel reactive antibody (PRA)
    II. HIV, hepatitis, herpes, Epstein Barr (EBV), herpes simplex, and cytomegalovirus
    III. Anti-citrullinated protein antibody (ACPA)
    IV. Toxoplasma and tuberculosis

    a. I and II
    b. I and IV
    c. I, III, and IV
    d. I, II, and IV

4. A kidney recipient presents with high fever, pain at surgical site, leukocytosis, renal allograft dysfunction, and urinary sediment. Which diagnostic test is indicated?

    a. Clean-catch midstream urine specimen for culture (bacterial and fungal)
    b. Catheterized urine specimen for culture
    c. Clean-catch midstream urine specimen for urinalysis
    d. Catheterized urine specimen for culture and blood culture

5. The age group that is most at risk for non-compliance with pre-cardiac transplantation and post-cardiac transplantation medical regimens and care is

    a. 65 to 75.
    b. 50 to 65.
    c. 25 to 50.
    d. 18 to 25.

6. Following heart transplantation, a decrease in the central venous pressure may be related to

    a. increased intravascular volume.
    b. cardiac tamponade.
    c. low intravascular volume.
    d. thrombus obstruction.

7. The average length of stay in the hospital for kidney transplant patients is

  a. 7 to 10 days.
  b. 12 to 14 days.
  c. 19 to 32 days.
  d. 55 to 72 days.

8. When educating a patient about the post-transplant complications, which of the following topics should be discussed?

  I. Infections
  II. Rejection
  III. Malignancies
  IV. Renal dysfunction

  a. I and II
  b. I, II, and IV
  c. I, II, and III
  d. I, II, III, and IV

9. Following heart transplantation, increased central venous pressure (CVP), distended neck veins, muffled heart sounds, and hypotension are indications of

  a. compartment syndrome.
  b. cardiac tamponade.
  c. disseminated intravascular coagulation (DIC).
  d. myocardial infarction.

10. If a lung recipient exhibits stridor and intermittent hypoxemia, which is resolved by coughing up sputum, the most likely diagnosis is

  a. primary graft dysfunction.
  b. inadequate bronchial anastomosis.
  c. pneumothorax.
  d. tracheobronchial stenosis.

11. Following a liver transplant, the initial laboratory indication of biliary obstruction is usually

  a. increased gamma glutamyltransferase (GGT).
  b. increased BUN and creatinine.
  c. increased serum alkaline phosphatase followed by increased bilirubin.
  d. increased bilirubin.

12. A pancreas transplant recipient experiencing an arterial thrombosis may exhibit an abrupt

  a. decrease in blood glucose.
  b. increase in blood glucose.
  c. decrease in serum amylase.
  d. increase in BUN.

13. Indications of low cardiac output in the heart recipient include

a. decreased BUN and serum creatinine.
b. metabolic alkalosis.
c. jugular venous distention.
d. hypertension.

14. Indications of acute tubular necrosis in a kidney recipient include

    I. increased BUN and creatinine.
    II. decreased BUN and creatinine.
    III. hypokalemia, hypophosphatemia, and hypomagnesemia.
    IV. pulmonary and peripheral edema.

a. I and IV
b. I, III, and IV
c. II, III, and IV
d. II and IV

15. When evaluating postoperative mediastinal bleeding, chest tube drainage should not exceed

a. 200 mL in 2 to 6 hours.
b. 300 mL in 1 to 3 hours.
c. 400 mL in 6 hours.
d. 500 mL in 4 hours.

16. A normal prothrombin time is

a. 21 to 35 seconds.
b. 10 to 15 seconds.
c. 30 to 45 seconds.
d. 2 to 9.5 minutes.

17. Which of the following effects are characteristic of Class II antidysrhythmic drugs, β-blockers (atenolol, esmolol, metoprolol)?

    I. Reduce SA nodal activity
    II. Block β-adrenergic cardiac stimulation
    III. Reduce ventricular contraction rate and cardiac output
    IV. Block both α- and β-adrenergic cardiac stimulation

a. I, III, and IV
b. II
c. I, II, and III
d. III and IV

18. The albumin value that indicates mild protein deficiency is

a. 3.5 to 5.5 g/dL.
b. 3 to 3.5 g/dL.
c. 2.5 to 3 g/dL.
d. <2.5 g/dL.

19. The pain management plan for a kidney recipient may include

a. fentanyl.
b. ibuprofen.
c. meperidine.
d. ketorolac.

20. Signs of kidney rejection include

a. weight increase, oliguria, jugular venous distention, irregular heartbeat, hypotension, fever, and dyspnea.
b. dyspnea, productive cough, fever, tiredness, and hypoxemia.
c. weight increase, increased BUN and creatinine, oliguria, peripheral edema, and fever.
d. abdominal pain or distention, nausea and vomiting, fever, change in stool output.

21. A patient is scheduled for a liver biopsy. Which of the following should be verified prior to the procedure?

   I. Coagulation test results
   II. Availability of donor blood
   III. Signed consent
   IV. Protein study results

a. I and III
b. I, III, and IV
c. I, II, and III
d. I, II, III, and IV

22. Following a liver biopsy, the correct positioning of the patient to prevent bleeding and bile peritonitis is

a. supine with only pressure dressing over biopsy site.
b. right-side lying with pressure dressing over biopsy site and pillow under the costal margin.
c. left-side lying with only pressure dressing in place over biopsy site.
d. prone with only pressure dressing in place over biopsy site.

23. Initial signs of pancreas rejection in a patient who received a pancreas transplant with a bladder-drained graft include

a. pain in right upper abdomen, increased serum amylase, and decreased urine amylase.
b. diffuse abdominal pain, decreased serum amylase, and increased urine amylase.
c. hyperglycemia, right upper abdomen pain, decreased serum amylase, and increased urine amylase.
d. hypoglycemia, diffuse abdominal pain, increased serum amylase, and decreased urine amylase.

24. Following heart transplant, infection of the deep soft tissue (including muscle and fascia) with purulent discharge and dehiscence along with fever, chills, local tenderness, chest wall pain, and unstable sternum is classified as

a. superficial infection.
b. sternal dehiscence.
c. sepsis.
d. mediastinitis.

25. A cardiac recipient exhibits ventricular arrhythmias with increasing changes in ECG, weakness with ascending paralysis and hyperreflexia, confusion, and diarrhea. Which of the following electrolyte imbalances do these signs and symptoms suggest?

    a. Hyperkalemia

    b. Hypokalemia

    c. Hypernatremia

    d. Hyponatremia

26. Adverse effects associated with calcineurin inhibitors include

    a. acne, weight gain, hypertension, osteoporosis, and cataracts.

    b. GI ulcerations and myelosuppression.

    c. hyperglycemia, neurotoxicity, and nephrotoxicity.

    d. elevated cholesterol and triglyceride levels and proteinuria.

27. Prior to administration of azathioprine to a renal transplant patient, which of the following must be assessed?

    a. Chest x-ray

    b. Platelet count and coagulation profile

    c. Vital signs, especially blood pressure and pulse

    d. CBC and lipid profile

28. Which of the following antifungal agents increases risk of nephrotoxicity when combined with tacrolimus or cyclosporine?

    a. Fluconazole

    b. Clotrimazole

    c. Amphotericin B

    d. Voriconazole

29. After teaching a patient incision care, the best technique to use to ensure the patient understands is

    a. ask the patient to give a return demonstration.

    b. give the patient a brief quiz.

    c. ask the patient to explain the procedure.

    d. provide written directions for the patient to refer to.

30. The most critical skill for a clinical transplant nurse collaborating in a transplant team is

    a. patience.

    b. assertiveness.

    c. empathy with others.

    d. willingness to compromise.

31. A necessary component of informed consent prior to a procedure is

    a. names of assisting staff members.

    b. beginning and ending times.

    c. risks and benefits of procedure.

    d. facility statistics regarding procedure.

32. Which of the following anti-ulcer agents may increase the risk of digoxin toxicity?

a. Omeprazole
b. Sucralfate
c. Cimetidine
d. Ranitidine

33. When preparing a patient for possible temporary hemodialysis after transplant, which of the following complications should the clinical transplant nurse review?

I. Hypotension and associated symptoms
II. Exsanguination
III. Muscle cramping
IV. Sleep disturbance

a. I, II, and IV
b. I, III, and IV
c. I
d. I and III

34. Under HIPAA guidelines, which of the following information can be communicated to a friend who is visiting a postoperative organ recipient?

a. Report of general condition
b. Detailed report of surgery
c. Prognosis
d. No information

35. The vaccination that is contraindicated in the post-transplant patient is

a. influenza.
b. measles-mumps-rubella.
c. pneumococcal.
d. tetanus.

36. A patient in renal failure hospitalized for transplant appears very upset after a physician's visit to discuss the transplantation. Which of the following is an example of therapeutic communication to encourage the patient to share feelings about the transplant/donor?

a. "Don't worry. Everything will be fine."
b. "You should trust your doctor."
c. "Is there anything you'd like to talk about?"
d. "Why are you so upset?"

37. The purpose of giving steroids (such as prednisone or methylprednisolone) in two divided doses, morning and afternoon, for pancreas recipients is to

a. control post-steroid hyperglycemia.
b. prevent GI symptoms.
c. reduce sodium and fluid retention.
d. reduce risk of fungal infections.

38. The therapeutic trough level for sirolimus during and following withdrawal from cyclosporine is

    a. 4 to 12 ng/mL.

    b. 12 to 24 ng/mL.

    c. 5 to 20 ng/mL.

    d. 3 to 8 ng/mL.

39. The primary target for transplant patients receiving statins, such as pravastatin, for hyperlipidemia is

    a. HDL level.

    b. triglyceride level.

    c. total cholesterol level.

    d. LDL level.

40. A patient with end-stage liver disease has a paracentesis to relieve massive ascites causing severe shortness of breath. Which of the following is used to reduce hyponatremia and renal dysfunction resulting from decreased effective arterial volume?

    a. Packed red blood cells

    b. Spironolactone

    c. Acetazolamide

    d. Albumin infusion

41. A patient with lung failure and severe shortness of breath is evaluated for lung transplantation. Which of the following is an absolute contraindication for lung transplantation?

    a. Age >55 for single-lung

    b. History of smoking within 12 months

    c. Corticosteroid dependency equivalent to >20 mg prednisone daily

    d. History of alcohol abuse

42. Following heart transplant, in the rewarming stage after hypothermia, a patient becomes hypotensive with decreased cardiac output because of vasodilation and hypovolemia. The usual initial treatment is

    a. bolus of 500 mL of lactated Ringers or NS.

    b. bolus of 500 mL of a colloid.

    c. blood transfusion.

    d. platelets.

43. Following a renal transplant, the patient's kidney is not yet functioning adequately but the patient is constipated. Which of the following laxatives/bowel control agents is contraindicated?

    a. Stool softener, such as Colace®

    b. Saline laxative, such as Milk of Magnesia®

    c. Bulk former, such as Metamucil®

    d. Lubricant, such as glycerine suppository

44. After liver transplant, a patient is receiving enteral feedings. Which of the following is the proper procedure to prevent occlusion of the feeding tube?

    a. Instill 5 to 10 mL of water over a minute and aspirate a number of times to flush each 8-hour period

    b. Flush with a 30 mL multi-enzyme cocktail of Pancrease and sodium bicarbonate solution every 4 hours

    c. Instill 30 mL of NS over a 5-minute period and aspirate to flush several times every 8 hours

    d. Flush with 30 mL of water every 4 hours and before and after feedings and medication administration

45. In the post-transplantation period, the patient's white blood count is 5300, but the absolute neutrophil count (ANC) is 526 mm³. The patient is at risk for

    a. bleeding.

    b. thromboembolia.

    c. no risk as WBC and ANC are normal.

    d. infection.

46. The transplant recipient is most at risk for cytomegalovirus (CMV) infection when

    a. donor and recipient both test positive for CMV.

    b. donor tests negative for CMV and recipient positive.

    c. donor and recipient both test negative for CMV.

    d. donor tests positive for CMV and recipient negative.

47. A patient receiving tacrolimus complains of pain in the mouth along with slight bleeding and loss of taste sensation. White lesions are evident on the mucosa. The most likely diagnosis is

    a. herpes simplex.

    b. gingivitis.

    c. oropharyngeal candidiasis.

    d. periodontitis.

48. The type of precautions indicated for a patient with a surgical site infection and purulent discharge is

    a. droplet.

    b. airborne.

    c. contact and droplet.

    d. contact.

49. A liver recipient is experiencing organ rejection. Which of the following agents is indicated for rejection that is already in progress?

    a. Mycophenolate mofetil

    b. Sirolimus

    c. Tacrolimus

    d. Muromonab-CD3

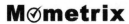

50. A patient is markedly neutropenic following immunosuppressive therapy. Which actions are included in measures to prevent infection?

I. Restrict fresh salads and unpeeled fresh fruit or vegetables from diet.

II. Provide patient with HEPA filter mask when patient is outside of room.

III. Change water in fresh flowers daily.

IV. Restrict visitors with illness, including colds or sore throats.

a. I and IV
b. I, II, and IV
c. I, II, III, and IV
d. I, III, and IV

Answer Key and Explanations

1. A: Metabolic abnormalities related to uremia include the following:

- Metabolic acidosis: Tubular cells are unable to regulate acid-base metabolism, and phosphate, sulfuric, hippuric, and lactic acids increase, leading to congestive heart failure and weakness.
- Decreased RBC production: Kidney is unable to produce adequate erythropoietin in peritubular cells, resulting in anemia, usually normocytic and normochromic. Parathyroid hormone levels may increase, causing bone marrow calcification, resulting in hypoproliferative anemia as RBC production is suppressed.
- Platelet abnormalities: Decreased platelet count, increased turnover, and reduced adhesion leads to bleeding disorders.
- Hyperkalemia: The nephrons cannot excrete adequate amounts of potassium. Some drugs, such as potassium-sparing diuretics, may aggravate the condition.

2. B: Short-acting regular insulin, such as Novolin R. Insulins include:

- Humalog (Lispro H): Rapid-acting, short duration insulin that acts within 5–15 minutes, peaking between 45–90 minutes and lasting 3–4 hours.
- NovoLog (aspart): Rapid-acting, short duration insulin, acting within 5–10 minutes, peaking in 1–3 hours, and lasting 3–5 hours.
- Regular (R) (Humulin R, Novolin R): Short-acting within 30 minutes, peaking in 2–5 hours, and lasting 5–8 hours.
- NPH (N): Intermediate–tracheostenosis
- Trach acting with onset in 1–3 hours, peaking at 6–12 hours (Humulin N) or 4–12 hours (Novolin N) and lasting 16–24 hours.
- Lantus (glargine): Long-acting insulin with onset in 1 hour and lasting 24 hours with no peak.

3. D: I, II, and IV. ABO blood typing, human leukocyte antigen (HLA), panel reactive antibody (PRA), HIV, hepatitis, herpes, Epstein Barr (EBV), herpes simplex, cytomegalovirus, toxoplasma, and tuberculosis screening is done pre-transplantation in addition to routine blood tests (such as CBC and differential and chem panel). Additionally, patients are screened for pre-existing cancers as immunosuppressive therapy, which increases risk of cancer, may interfere with cancer treatment. Post-menopausal women are also assessed for osteoporosis as immunosuppressive agents increase risk of bone loss.

4. A: High fever, pain at surgical site, leukocytosis, renal allograft dysfunction, and urinary sediment are consistent with urinary tract infection, such as pyelonephritis. A clean-catch midstream urine specimen should be obtained for culture (bacterial and fungal). Treatment depends on the results of the culture and sensitivities although treatment may begin with TMP-SMX or fluoroquinolones, which may also be used prophylactically to prevent infection. Routine urine cultures should be obtained after kidney transplant for surveillance purposes.

5. D: Those who are 18 to 25 have the lowest survival rates and are most at risk for non-compliance because young adults are establishing their independence and identities and may have difficulty following through with medications and appointments and may be especially stressed by alterations in self-image or peer approval. They may have school or work-related demands that interfere with treatment. Additionally, following surgery, as patients begin to feel better, they may feel unrealistically that they are completely healthy and don't need treatment.

6. C: Decreased CVP is related to low intravascular volume, decreased preload, or vasodilation. Hemodynamic monitoring is the monitoring of blood flow pressures. In order for effective post-surgical cardiac functioning, the correct relationship between high and low pressures must be maintained. Central venous pressure (CVP), the pressure in the right atrium or vena cava, is used to assess function of the right ventricles, preload, and flow of venous blood to the heart. Normal pressure ranges from 2–5 mm Hg but may be elevated after surgery to 6–8 mm Hg. Incorrect catheter placement or malfunctioning can affect readings.

7. A: Length of stay varies according to the patient's condition and type of transplant, but the usual length of stay for kidney transplant patients is about 7 to 10 days (average 8.6). Liver transplant patients usually have a longer stay, averaging 12 to 14 days while the cardiac transplant patient's length of stays has a wider range of 19 to 32 days. Patients receiving small intestine transplants may require about 55 days of hospitalization and up to 72 days if receiving multivisceral transplants.

8. D: Infections, rejection, malignancies, and renal dysfunction are all common complications of transplantation and should be covered in patient education. Infection is a high risk after surgery because of immunosuppressive drugs, and patients must be monitored carefully and taught signs of infection. Compliance with treatment regimen is critical to preventing organ rejection. Malignancies may occur as a long-term complication of immunosuppression. Renal dysfunction often occurs as the result of hypovolemia, infection, or drugs that impair renal function, such as calcineurin inhibitors.

9. B: Beck's triad (distended neck veins, muffled heart sounds, and hypotension) and increased CVP are indicative of cardiac tamponade. A sudden decrease in chest tube drainage can occur as fluid and clots accumulate in the pericardial sac, preventing the blood from filling the ventricles and decreasing cardiac output and perfusion of the body, including the kidneys (resulting in decreased urinary output). About 50 ml of fluid normally circulates in the pericardial area to reduce friction. A sudden increase in volume can compress the heart, causing a number of cardiac responses:

- Increased end-diastolic pressure in both ventricles.
- Decreased venous return.
- Decreased ventricular filling.

10. D: Stridor and intermittent hypoxemia, which are resolved by coughing up sputum, are characteristic of tracheobronchial stenosis. On palpation, a tracheal rumble may be noted for tracheal stenosis. Bronchial stenosis is most common and may occur at the site of anastomosis or distal to the site. The patient should have an emergent bronchoscopy to confirm diagnosis. CT may be done to show luminal diameter on inspiration and expiration. Treatment may include corticosteroids (high dose) and balloon dilation or stenting.

11. C: The initial laboratory indication of biliary obstruction is increased serum alkaline phosphatase (normal value = 20–125 U/L) followed by increased bilirubin level. Obstruction is usually related to complications with the anastomosis. Diagnostic procedures include an ultrasound, which may show biliary dilation but is not diagnostic if dilation is absent, and cholangiography to confirm. Magnetic resonance cholangiopancreatography (MRCP) has a high sensitivity for diagnosis. Early obstruction usually occurs at the site of duct-to-duct reconstruction (choledochocholedochostomy [CDCD]).

12. B: A pancreas transplant recipient experiencing an arterial thrombosis may exhibit an abrupt increase in blood glucose levels while serum amylase levels remain relatively stable. Vascular thrombosis may be venous (most common) or arterial and usually occurs within the first 24 to 48 hours after transplantation. Patients usually receive some type of anticoagulation therapy or a combination of anticoagulation therapy and antiplatelet therapy as prophylaxis, such as IV heparin, enoxaparin, and aspirin. Careful handling of the organ during the procurement procedures may help prevent this complication.

13. C: Jugular venous distention is a sign of low cardiac output. Other signs and symptoms include dysrhythmias, cyanosis, pallor, cool clammy skin, impaired capillary refill, increased serum creatinine and BUN, oliguria/anuria, tachypnea, dyspnea, metabolic acidosis, basilar crackles, and mental status changes. Treatment may include atrial or AV sequential pacing, volume infusion, blood products, vasopressors, inotropes and anti-rejection agents. Circulatory support, such as with an IABP, may be required for graft failure. Causes may include decreased heart rate, hypovolemia, third space fluid shift, increased systemic vascular resistance, cardiac tamponade, dysrhythmias, graft failure, and rejection.

14. A: I and IV. Acute tubular necrosis (ATN) occurs when a hypoxic condition causes renal ischemia that damages tubular cells of the glomeruli so they are unable to adequately filter the urine, leading to acute renal failure. Indications include increased BUN and creatinine, hyperkalemia, hyperphosphatemia, hypermagnesemia, and pulmonary and peripheral edema. Urinary sediment is tubular epithelial or granular. Patients may exhibit lethargy and nausea and vomiting. ATN can result in uremia, leading to destruction of platelets and bleeding, neurological deficits, and disseminated intravascular coagulopathy (DIC).

15. A: Chest tube drainage should not exceed 200 mL in 2 to 6 hours. Acute onset of bleeding is characterized by bright red blood and continuous steady discharge. Dark red blood suggests older blood rather than active bleeding, especially if discharge slows after initial increase. Bleeding may be surgical (bleeding from vessel or sutures) or nonsurgical (related to coagulopathy). Indications for emergent surgical exploration include:

- Blood loss >400 mL/hr X 4 hours.
- Blood loss 300 mL/hr X 3 hours.
- Blood loss 400 mL/hr X 2 hours.
- Blood loss 500 mL/hr X 1 hour.

16. B:

Prothrombin time (PT)	10–15 seconds	Increases with anticoagulation therapy, vitamin K deficiency, decreased prothrombin, DIC, liver disease, and malignant neoplasm.
Partial thromboplastin time (PTT)	30–45 seconds	Increases with hemophilia A & B, von Willebrand's, vitamin K deficiency, lupus, DIC, and liver disease.
Activated partial thromboplastin time (aPTT)	21–35 seconds	Similar to PTT, but decreases in extensive cancer, early DIC, and after acute hemorrhage. Used to monitor heparin dosage.
Thrombin clotting time (TCT) or Thrombin time (TT)	7–12 seconds (<21)	Used most often to determine dosage of heparin.
Bleeding time	2–9.5 minutes	Increases with DIC, leukemia, renal failure, aplastic anemia, von Willebrand's, some drugs, and alcohol.
Platelet count	150–400,000	Increased bleeding <50,000 and increased clotting >750,000.

17. C: I, II, and III. β-adrenergic blockers block sympathetic nervous stimulation of the heart, thereby reducing SA nodal activity and atrial ectopic foci stimulation. They reduce the ventricular contraction rate and cardiac output, reducing blood pressure. β-adrenergic blockers are used primarily to control angina and hypertension and to treat supraventricular and ventricular dysrhythmias. β-blockers may interact with numerous other medications, with some reducing β-blocker activity (antacids, NSAIDS, rifampin, ampicillin, phenothiazines) and others enhancing activity (cimetidine, loop diuretics, other antidysrhythmics).

18. B: Albumin is a protein that is produced by the liver and is a necessary component for cells and tissues. Albumin levels are the most common screening to determine protein levels. Albumin has a half-life of 18–20 days, so it is sensitive to long-term protein deficiencies more than short-term:

- Normal values: 3.5 to 5.5 g/dL
- Mild deficiency: 3 to 3.5 g/dL
- Moderate deficiency: 2.5 to 3.0 g/dL
- Severe deficiency: <2.5 g/dL.

Levels below 3.2 correlate with increased morbidity and death. Dehydration (poor intake, diarrhea, or vomiting) elevates levels, so adequate hydration is important to ensure meaningful results.

19. A: After kidney transplant, patient-controlled analgesia is commonly used with morphine or fentanyl for the first 24 to 48 hours, after which patients can usually be maintained with oxycodone or propoxyphene. Meperidine should be avoided because it depends on the kidneys to excrete metabolites, which can be retained because the new kidney is limited in function, resulting in seizures. NSAIDS, such as ibuprofen and ketorolac, may impair renal perfusion as well as increase the risk of bleeding.

20. C: Signs of kidney rejection include weight increase, increased BUN and creatinine, oliguria, peripheral edema, and fever as well as general malaise and fatigue and increased pain at operative site. Rejection is classified as hyperacute, accelerated, acute, and chronic, based on etiology, T-cell (most common) or B-cell mediated, and onset of symptoms:

- Hyperacute: Immediately after surgery.
- Accelerated: 24 hours to 5 days after surgery.
- Acute: A few days to weeks after surgery.
- Chronic: Months to years after surgery.

21. C: Liver biopsy requires removal of a small amount of tissue, usually through needle aspiration. Coagulation studies should be obtained prior to the procedure and abnormalities treated as bleeding is a major complication. Additionally, donor blood should be available in the event of bleeding. Informed consent must always be obtained before invasive procedures. Protein studies are not required for liver biopsy. The patient's vital signs should also be taken prior to the procedure to serve as a baseline to evaluate changes.

22. B: Following a liver biopsy, the patient should be positioned on the right side with a pressure dressing over the biopsy site and a pillow under the costal margin as this position compresses the liver capsule at the insertion site against the chest wall, preventing bleeding and escape of bile through the needle insertion site. Vital signs should be checked every 10 to 15 minutes for an hour and then every half hour for 1 to 2 hours or until the patient's condition is stable. The patient should be advised to restrict activities and lifting for a week.

23. A: Initial signs of pancreas rejection in a patient who received a pancreas transplant with a bladder-drained graft include pain in right upper abdomen, increased serum amylase, and decreased urine amylase. Symptoms are often very non-specific although hyperglycemia is usually a late sign as glucose levels remain within normal limits initially. A biopsy is required to confirm rejection, after which patients should be kept on bedrest and observed for signs of bleeding or hematoma. Treatment for pancreas rejection may include IV pulse steroids and antilymphocyte agents.

24. D: Mediastinitis (Type 3): Infection of the deep soft tissue (including muscle and fascia) with purulent discharge and dehiscence along with fever, chills, local tenderness, chest wall pain, and unstable sternum. Superficial infection (Type 1): Cellulitis, with local tenderness, erythema, and serous drainage. Small areas of wound breakdown may occur with some purulent discharge. Sternal dehiscence (Type 2): Usually associated with coagulase-negative staphylococcus and *Staphylococcus aureus* and classified into 3 categories:

- Bone is sterile and viable.
- Sternal osteitis present in proximal two-thirds of sternum with non-viable bone.
- Sternal osteitis present in distal third of sternum with non-viable bone.

25. A: Hyperkalemia (>5.5 mEq/L, critical value: >6.5 mEq/L) can result from high-potassium cardioplegic solutions, low cardiac output with oliguria, tissue ischemia, acute/chronic renal insufficiency, and medications (ARBs, NSAIDs, β-blockers, ACEIs, K-sparing diuretics). The primary symptoms relate to the effect on the cardiac muscle:

- Ventricular arrhythmias with increasing changes in EKG leading to cardiac and respiratory arrest.
- Weakness with ascending paralysis and hyperreflexia.
- Diarrhea.
- Increasing confusion.

26. C: Adverse effects of calcineurin inhibitors (cyclosporine, tacrolimus) include hyperglycemia, neurotoxicity, nephrotoxicity, diabetes mellitus, and hypertension. Neurotoxicity may result in headaches, tremor, and seizures. Cyclosporine may also cause hyperlipidemia and hirsutism while tacrolimus is associated with electrolyte imbalances, including hyperkalemia, hypophosphatemia and hypomagnesemia. Calcineurin inhibitors must be used with care in combination with other drugs as some drugs, such as antifungal agents, CCBs, and macrolide antibiotics, potentiate action by increasing drug concentration, and others, such as anti-epileptic agents and some antibiotics (nafcillin, rifampin, and rifabutin), decrease drug concentration.

27. B: Because azathioprine is associated with thrombocytopenia, the platelet count and coagulation profile should be assessed. Other adverse effects include leukopenia and hepatotoxicity. Azathioprine is an immunosuppressant agent that blocks purine metabolism, inhibiting the synthesis of T-cell DNA, RNA, and proteins, which blocks the normal immune response. Azathioprine is used to prevent organ rejection in renal transplantation. Azathioprine may be administered orally or intravenously. Azathioprine should not be given with allopurinol, which interferes with azathioprine's metabolism, potentiating its effects. Giving azathioprine with ACE inhibitors may cause severe leukopenia, and azathioprine may reduce effectiveness of anticoagulants.

28. C: Amphotericin B increases risk of nephrotoxicity when combined with cyclosporine or tacrolimus. Amphotericin B is used to treat candidiasis, blastomycosis, aspergillosis, coccidioidomycosis, cryptococcosis, leishmaniasis, and sporotrichosis. Other adverse effects include hypokalemia and hypomagnesemia and elevated liver enzymes. Almost all patients receiving IV amphotericin B experience flu-like symptoms with fever, chills, malaise, muscle/joint aching, hypotension, tachycardia, headache, nausea and vomiting, so antipyretics, antihistamines, and antiemetics may be given concurrently. Lipid preparations are also available. Because side effects may be severe, a 1-mg test dose may be given over a 20- to 30-minute period to determine the patient's tolerance for the drug.

29. A: A return demonstration is given by patients to show mastery of a procedure. This may be done for each step during initial instruction but should eventually include a demonstration of the entire procedure:

- The nurse should ask if the patient has any questions before the demonstration.
- The patient should gather all necessary equipment, using a checklist to ensure that nothing is forgotten.
- The patient should explain the steps.
- The nurse should provide positive feedback occasionally during the procedure: "You've placed the equipment exactly right," and may remind the patient to look at the checklist.

30. D: While all of these characteristics are important for team members, central to collaboration is the willingness to compromise. In addition, members must be able to communicate clearly, which encompasses assertiveness, patience, and empathy. Teams should identify specific challenges and problems and then focus on the task of reaching a solution. Collaboration is needed in order to move nursing forward. Nurses must take an active role in gathering data for evidence-based practice to support nursing's role in health care and must share this information with other nurses and health professionals.

31. C: Patients/family should be apprised of all reasonable risks and any complications that might be life threatening or increase morbidity, as well as benefits. The American Medical Association has established guidelines for informed consent:

- Explanation of diagnosis.
- Nature and reason for treatment or procedure.
- Risks and benefits.
- Alternative options (regardless of cost or insurance coverage).
- Risks and benefits of alternative options.
- Risks and benefits of not having a treatment or procedure.
- Providing informed consent is a requirement of all states.

32. A: Omeprazole and other proton pump inhibitors may increase absorption of digoxin and increase risk of toxicity. PPIs also may increase INR in those on warfarin and decrease the absorption of the antifungals ketoconazole and itraconazole. PPIs block over 90% of gastric acid secretion over 24 hours. Omeprazole is indicated for esophagitis, duodenal ulcer (*H. pylori* infections), NSAID-induced ulcers, reflux, and hypersecretory conditions. Adverse effects include diarrhea, abdominal discomfort, flatulence, nausea, vomiting, headache, dizziness, and vertigo.

33. B: I, III, and IV. The clinical transplant nurse should prepare the patient for complications that he or she may experience directly (hypotension, muscle cramping, and sleep disturbance) and help the person learn strategies to recognize these complications and deal with them. Exsanguination can occur if blood lines separate or dialysis needles become dislodged during hemodialysis, but preventing these types of complications is the responsibility of the professional staff. If the patient is to have long-term dialysis at home, then teaching about the possibility of exsanguination becomes important.

34. D: No information can be provided without explicit permission of the patient. The Health Insurance Portability and Accountability Act (HIPAA) addresses the rights of the individual related to privacy of health information. The clinical transplant nurse must not release any information or documentation about a patient's condition or treatment without consent, as the individual has the right to determine who has access to personal information. Personal information about the patient is considered protected health information (PHI), and consists of any identifying or personal information such as health history, condition, or treatments in any form, and any documentation.

35. B: Live-attenuated vaccines such as MMR, oral polio, and varicella are contraindicated in organ recipients because viral replication may occur in those immunocompromised. Additionally, household members should also avoid this type of vaccination. Post-transplant patients usually are advised to get yearly influenza vaccinations, pneumococcal vaccinations every 5 to 6 years, and tetanus boosters every 10 years; however, vaccines may be less effective. Pre-transplant adults are usually advised to be vaccinated for hepatitis A and B, *S. pneumoniae,* tetanus, influenza, and varicella.

36. C: "Is there anything you'd like to talk about?" is an open-ended question that encourages the patient to share feelings. Other examples of therapeutic communications are statements that show empathy and observations such as "You are shaking" or "You seem worried." Clinical transplant nurses should avoid providing advice ("should" or "must") and avoid meaningless clichés, such as "Don't worry. Everything will be fine." Asking for explanations of behavior not directly related to patient care, such as "Why are you so upset?" should also be avoided.

37. A: Because corticosteroids can cause hyperglycemia, pancreas recipients who are prescribed steroids may receive the drug in two divided doses, morning and afternoon. Other adverse effects include hypokalemia and hypernatremia, mood changes, headaches, vertigo, Cushing's syndrome, hypothalamic-pituitary-adrenal axis suppression, GI upset and ulcers, hirsutism, skin fragility, petechiae, muscle weakness, osteoporosis, glaucoma, cataracts, and weight gain. Steroids may mask symptoms of bacterial or fungal infections. Concurrent use with non–potassium-sparing diuretics may lead to hypocalcemia and hypokalemia.

38. B: The therapeutic trough level for sirolimus during and following withdrawal from cyclosporine is 12 to 24 ng/mL in whole blood. This is higher than the normal therapeutic target of 4 to 12 ng/mL. Trough levels should be evaluated about 4 or 5 days after a change in dosage. Trough level refers to the lowest concentration of the agent in the body after levels fall from the peak level. Trough levels should be monitored carefully and dosage adjusted to obtain optimal levels.

39. D: The primary target for transplant patients receiving statins is the LDL level.

LDL cholesterol	< 100 = Optimal 100– 129 = Near optimal 130– 159 = Borderline high 160– 189 = High ≥190 = Very high
Total cholesterol	< 200 = Optimal 200– 239 = Borderline high ≥240 = High
HDL cholesterol	< 40 = Low ≥60 = High (optimal)
Triglycerides	< 150 = Normal 150– 199 = Borderline – high 200– 499 = High ≥500 = Very high

40. D: Albumin infusions are used to reduce hyponatremia and renal dysfunction resulting from decreased effective arterial volume after paracentesis. Paracentesis is usually done only to relieve severe symptoms, such as shortness of breath, after sodium restriction and use of diuretics (usually spironolactone) have proven ineffective. Spironolactone helps to prevent potassium loss. Other diuretics, such as furosemide, may be added but must be carefully monitored as severe hyponatremia may result. Acetazolamide is contraindicated because it increases risk of hepatic coma.

41. C: Corticosteroid dependency equivalent to >20 mg prednisone daily is an absolute contraindication for lung transplantation. Other contraindications include age >65 for single lung, >55 for bilateral lung, and >45 for heart-lung transplants. Patients should have no history of smoking for 6 months and no current alcohol, drug, or tobacco abuse. Patients must be emotionally stable and able to understand and comply with medical regimens and have a psychosocial support system. Body weight should not exceed 140% of predicted or be less than 80% of predicted.

42. A: The usual initial bolus of fluid is 500 mL of lactated Ringers or NS. Colloids should be avoided with capillary leak syndrome but are indicated for hypotension primarily related to peripheral vasodilation. Volume resuscitation must be adequate to maintain filling pressures, especially in the first 6 postoperative hours, but overloading the patient with fluid (>2L/6 hrs) may result in hemodilution, requiring blood transfusions and plasma or platelets to increase clotting factors and prevent bleeding.

43. B: People with impairment of kidney function should avoid products containing magnesium or phosphates, which can cause acute phosphate nephropathy. Saline laxatives, such as Milk of Magnesia® and Epsom salt, contain ions, such as magnesium phosphate, magnesium hydroxide, and citrate, which are not absorbed through the intestines and draw more fluid into the stool. The magnesium in the preparations also stimulates the bowel. Stool softeners, bulk formers, and lubricants, such as glycerine suppositories, are usually well tolerated but bulk formers may result in constipation if fluid intake is inadequate.

44. D: Prevention of occlusion involves proper administration of medications and feedings, and maintaining a regular schedule of flushing. Tubes should be flushed with 30 ml of water at least every 4 hours as well as before and after feedings and administration of medications. Medications should be in liquid form or crushed completely, and enteric-coated or delayed-release preparations should be avoided. Feeding solutions should be liquid consistency. Patient should be positioned with head elevated for feedings.

45. D: While the patient's white blood count is within normal parameters, the normal absolute neutrophil count (ANC) for an adult is 1800 to 7700 mm^3. The risk of infection increases markedly if the ANC falls below 1000 mm^3 and is severe at <500 mm^3. A drop in the ANC leads to the condition of neutropenia, a severe complication of immunosuppression. Neutropenia increases risk of both exogenous and endogenous infection. Patients with both neutropenia and a fever usually have an infection that could quickly become life threatening.

46. D: Highest risk (up to 60%) occurs when the donor tests positive for CMV and the recipient tests negative. When both the donor and recipient test positive or the donor tests negative and the recipient positive, the risk is moderate (20–40%). The lowest risk occurs when both the donor and recipient test negative, but the recipient may develop primary CMV from community exposure or contaminated blood. Lung and small bowel recipients have the highest risk for development of CMV with moderate risk to those receiving liver, pancreas, and heart, and low risk to kidney recipients.

47. C: Pain in the mouth, slight bleeding, loss of taste sensation, and white lesions on the mucosa are consistent with oropharyngeal candidiasis (thrush), caused by the *Candida albicans* fungus. Treatment can include nystatin oral suspension and clotrimazole although clotrimazole may cause hepatotoxicity. Amphotericin B should be avoided with nephrotoxic drugs such as tacrolimus. Transplant patients may be treated with prophylactic antifungals to prevent candidiasis. Candidiasis must be treated as it can spread systemically in those who are immunosuppressed.

48. D: Contact precautions.

Contact	Use personal protective equipment (PPE), including gown and gloves, for all contacts with the patient or patient's immediate environment. Maintain patient in private room or >3 feet away from other patients.
Droplet	(Appropriate for influenza, streptococcus infection, pertussis, rhinovirus, and adenovirus and pathogens that remain viable and infectious for only short distances.) Use mask while caring for the patient. Maintain patient in a private room or >3 feet away from other patients with curtain separating them. Use patient mask if transporting patient from one area to another.
Airborne	(Appropriate for measles, chickenpox, tuberculosis, and SARS because pathogens remain viable and infectious for long distances.) Place patient in an airborne infection isolation room. Use N95 respirators (or masks) while caring for patient.

49. D: While a number of drugs are used to prevent rejection, muromonab-CD3 is indicated to treat acute organ rejection that is already in progress. It is used for acute rejection of kidney, liver, and heart transplants. Muromonab-CD3 binds to CD3 glycoprotein on receptors in T-cells, blocking antigen recognition. Adverse effects include chest pain, fever, chills, tremor, vomiting, nausea, diarrhea, dyspnea, wheezing, pulmonary edema, and fluid retention.

50. B: I, II, and IV. Fresh vegetables and fruits may harbor bacteria, so salads and unpeeled fresh fruit or vegetables should be restricted from the neutropenic diet. Patients with ANC <1000 should be placed in private rooms and use HEPA filters if leaving the room. Visitors with any type of contagious illness should be restricted. Fresh flowers are prohibited because stagnant water can breed bacteria. Fluids in all other containers, including humidifiers, should be changed daily. Patients should be provided good oral care and personal hygiene.

How to Overcome Test Anxiety

Just the thought of taking a test is enough to make most people a little nervous. A test is an important event that can have a long-term impact on your future, so it's important to take it seriously and it's natural to feel anxious about performing well. But just because anxiety is normal, that doesn't mean that it's helpful in test taking, or that you should simply accept it as part of your life. Anxiety can have a variety of effects. These effects can be mild, like making you feel slightly nervous, or severe, like blocking your ability to focus or remember even a simple detail.

If you experience test anxiety—whether severe or mild—it's important to know how to beat it. To discover this, first you need to understand what causes test anxiety.

Causes of Test Anxiety

While we often think of anxiety as an uncontrollable emotional state, it can actually be caused by simple, practical things. One of the most common causes of test anxiety is that a person does not feel adequately prepared for their test. This feeling can be the result of many different issues such as poor study habits or lack of organization, but the most common culprit is time management. Starting to study too late, failing to organize your study time to cover all of the material, or being distracted while you study will mean that you're not well prepared for the test. This may lead to cramming the night before, which will cause you to be physically and mentally exhausted for the test. Poor time management also contributes to feelings of stress, fear, and hopelessness as you realize you are not well prepared but don't know what to do about it.

Other times, test anxiety is not related to your preparation for the test but comes from unresolved fear. This may be a past failure on a test, or poor performance on tests in general. It may come from comparing yourself to others who seem to be performing better or from the stress of living up to expectations. Anxiety may be driven by fears of the future—how failure on this test would affect your educational and career goals. These fears are often completely irrational, but they can still negatively impact your test performance.

Review Video: 3 Reasons You Have Test Anxiety
Visit mometrix.com/academy and enter code: 428468

107

Elements of Test Anxiety

As mentioned earlier, test anxiety is considered to be an emotional state, but it has physical and mental components as well. Sometimes you may not even realize that you are suffering from test anxiety until you notice the physical symptoms. These can include trembling hands, rapid heartbeat, sweating, nausea, and tense muscles. Extreme anxiety may lead to fainting or vomiting. Obviously, any of these symptoms can have a negative impact on testing. It is important to recognize them as soon as they begin to occur so that you can address the problem before it damages your performance.

Review Video: 3 Ways to Tell You Have Test Anxiety
Visit mometrix.com/academy and enter code: 927847

The mental components of test anxiety include trouble focusing and inability to remember learned information. During a test, your mind is on high alert, which can help you recall information and stay focused for an extended period of time. However, anxiety interferes with your mind's natural processes, causing you to blank out, even on the questions you know well. The strain of testing during anxiety makes it difficult to stay focused, especially on a test that may take several hours. Extreme anxiety can take a huge mental toll, making it difficult not only to recall test information but even to understand the test questions or pull your thoughts together.

Review Video: How Test Anxiety Affects Memory
Visit mometrix.com/academy and enter code: 609003

Effects of Test Anxiety

Test anxiety is like a disease—if left untreated, it will get progressively worse. Anxiety leads to poor performance, and this reinforces the feelings of fear and failure, which in turn lead to poor performances on subsequent tests. It can grow from a mild nervousness to a crippling condition. If allowed to progress, test anxiety can have a big impact on your schooling, and consequently on your future.

Test anxiety can spread to other parts of your life. Anxiety on tests can become anxiety in any stressful situation, and blanking on a test can turn into panicking in a job situation. But fortunately, you don't have to let anxiety rule your testing and determine your grades. There are a number of relatively simple steps you can take to move past anxiety and function normally on a test and in the rest of life.

Review Video: How Test Anxiety Impacts Your Grades
Visit mometrix.com/academy and enter code: 939819

Physical Steps for Beating Test Anxiety

While test anxiety is a serious problem, the good news is that it can be overcome. It doesn't have to control your ability to think and remember information. While it may take time, you can begin taking steps today to beat anxiety.

Just as your first hint that you may be struggling with anxiety comes from the physical symptoms, the first step to treating it is also physical. Rest is crucial for having a clear, strong mind. If you are tired, it is much easier to give in to anxiety. But if you establish good sleep habits, your body and mind will be ready to perform optimally, without the strain of exhaustion. Additionally, sleeping well helps you to retain information better, so you're more likely to recall the answers when you see the test questions.

Getting good sleep means more than going to bed on time. It's important to allow your brain time to relax. Take study breaks from time to time so it doesn't get overworked, and don't study right before bed. Take time to rest your mind before trying to rest your body, or you may find it difficult to fall asleep.

Review Video: The Importance of Sleep for Your Brain
Visit mometrix.com/academy and enter code: 319338

Along with sleep, other aspects of physical health are important in preparing for a test. Good nutrition is vital for good brain function. Sugary foods and drinks may give a burst of energy but this burst is followed by a crash, both physically and emotionally. Instead, fuel your body with protein and vitamin-rich foods.

Also, drink plenty of water. Dehydration can lead to headaches and exhaustion, especially if your brain is already under stress from the rigors of the test. Particularly if your test is a long one, drink water during the breaks. And if possible, take an energy-boosting snack to eat between sections.

Review Video: How Diet Can Affect your Mood
Visit mometrix.com/academy and enter code: 624317

Along with sleep and diet, a third important part of physical health is exercise. Maintaining a steady workout schedule is helpful, but even taking 5-minute study breaks to walk can help get your blood pumping faster and clear your head. Exercise also releases endorphins, which contribute to a positive feeling and can help combat test anxiety.

When you nurture your physical health, you are also contributing to your mental health. If your body is healthy, your mind is much more likely to be healthy as well. So take time to rest, nourish your body with healthy food and water, and get moving as much as possible. Taking these physical steps will make you stronger and more able to take the mental steps necessary to overcome test anxiety.

Review Video: How to Stay Healthy and Prevent Test Anxiety
Visit mometrix.com/academy and enter code: 877894

Mental Steps for Beating Test Anxiety

Working on the mental side of test anxiety can be more challenging, but as with the physical side, there are clear steps you can take to overcome it. As mentioned earlier, test anxiety often stems from lack of preparation, so the obvious solution is to prepare for the test. Effective studying may be the most important weapon you have for beating test anxiety, but you can and should employ several other mental tools to combat fear.

First, boost your confidence by reminding yourself of past success—tests or projects that you aced. If you're putting as much effort into preparing for this test as you did for those, there's no reason you should expect to fail here. Work hard to prepare; then trust your preparation.

Second, surround yourself with encouraging people. It can be helpful to find a study group, but be sure that the people you're around will encourage a positive attitude. If you spend time with others who are anxious or cynical, this will only contribute to your own anxiety. Look for others who are motivated to study hard from a desire to succeed, not from a fear of failure.

Third, reward yourself. A test is physically and mentally tiring, even without anxiety, and it can be helpful to have something to look forward to. Plan an activity following the test, regardless of the outcome, such as going to a movie or getting ice cream.

When you are taking the test, if you find yourself beginning to feel anxious, remind yourself that you know the material. Visualize successfully completing the test. Then take a few deep, relaxing breaths and return to it. Work through the questions carefully but with confidence, knowing that you are capable of succeeding.

Developing a healthy mental approach to test taking will also aid in other areas of life. Test anxiety affects more than just the actual test—it can be damaging to your mental health and even contribute to depression. It's important to beat test anxiety before it becomes a problem for more than testing.

Review Video: Test Anxiety and Depression
Visit mometrix.com/academy and enter code: 904704

Study Strategy

Being prepared for the test is necessary to combat anxiety, but what does being prepared look like? You may study for hours on end and still not feel prepared. What you need is a strategy for test prep. The next few pages outline our recommended steps to help you plan out and conquer the challenge of preparation.

STEP 1: SCOPE OUT THE TEST

Learn everything you can about the format (multiple choice, essay, etc.) and what will be on the test. Gather any study materials, course outlines, or sample exams that may be available. Not only will this help you to prepare, but knowing what to expect can help to alleviate test anxiety.

STEP 2: MAP OUT THE MATERIAL

Look through the textbook or study guide and make note of how many chapters or sections it has. Then divide these over the time you have. For example, if a book has 15 chapters and you have five days to study, you need to cover three chapters each day. Even better, if you have the time, leave an extra day at the end for overall review after you have gone through the material in depth.

If time is limited, you may need to prioritize the material. Look through it and make note of which sections you think you already have a good grasp on, and which need review. While you are studying, skim quickly through the familiar sections and take more time on the challenging parts. Write out your plan so you don't get lost as you go. Having a written plan also helps you feel more in control of the study, so anxiety is less likely to arise from feeling overwhelmed at the amount to cover.

STEP 3: GATHER YOUR TOOLS

Decide what study method works best for you. Do you prefer to highlight in the book as you study and then go back over the highlighted portions? Or do you type out notes of the important information? Or is it helpful to make flashcards that you can carry with you? Assemble the pens, index cards, highlighters, post-it notes, and any other materials you may need so you won't be distracted by getting up to find things while you study.

If you're having a hard time retaining the information or organizing your notes, experiment with different methods. For example, try color-coding by subject with colored pens, highlighters, or post-it notes. If you learn better by hearing, try recording yourself reading your notes so you can listen while in the car, working out, or simply sitting at your desk. Ask a friend to quiz you from your flashcards, or try teaching someone the material to solidify it in your mind.

STEP 4: CREATE YOUR ENVIRONMENT

It's important to avoid distractions while you study. This includes both the obvious distractions like visitors and the subtle distractions like an uncomfortable chair (or a too-comfortable couch that makes you want to fall asleep). Set up the best study environment possible: good lighting and a comfortable work area. If background music helps you focus, you may want to turn it on, but otherwise keep the room quiet. If you are using a computer to take notes, be sure you don't have any other windows open, especially applications like social media, games, or anything else that could distract you. Silence your phone and turn off notifications. Be sure to keep water close by so you stay hydrated while you study (but avoid unhealthy drinks and snacks).

Also, take into account the best time of day to study. Are you freshest first thing in the morning? Try to set aside some time then to work through the material. Is your mind clearer in the afternoon or evening? Schedule your study session then. Another method is to study at the same time of day that you will take the test, so that your brain gets used to working on the material at that time and will be ready to focus at test time.

STEP 5: STUDY!

Once you have done all the study preparation, it's time to settle into the actual studying. Sit down, take a few moments to settle your mind so you can focus, and begin to follow your study plan. Don't give in to distractions or let yourself procrastinate. This is your time to prepare so you'll be ready to fearlessly approach the test. Make the most of the time and stay focused.

Of course, you don't want to burn out. If you study too long you may find that you're not retaining the information very well. Take regular study breaks. For example, taking five minutes out of every hour to walk briskly, breathing deeply and swinging your arms, can help your mind stay fresh.

As you get to the end of each chapter or section, it's a good idea to do a quick review. Remind yourself of what you learned and work on any difficult parts. When you feel that you've mastered the material, move on to the next part. At the end of your study session, briefly skim through your notes again.

But while review is helpful, cramming last minute is NOT. If at all possible, work ahead so that you won't need to fit all your study into the last day. Cramming overloads your brain with more information than it can process and retain, and your tired mind may struggle to recall even previously learned information when it is overwhelmed with last-minute study. Also, the urgent nature of cramming and the stress placed on your brain contribute to anxiety. You'll be more likely to go to the test feeling unprepared and having trouble thinking clearly.

So don't cram, and don't stay up late before the test, even just to review your notes at a leisurely pace. Your brain needs rest more than it needs to go over the information again. In fact, plan to finish your studies by noon or early afternoon the day before the test. Give your brain the rest of the day to relax or focus on other things, and get a good night's sleep. Then you will be fresh for the test and better able to recall what you've studied.

STEP 6: TAKE A PRACTICE TEST

Many courses offer sample tests, either online or in the study materials. This is an excellent resource to check whether you have mastered the material, as well as to prepare for the test format and environment.

Check the test format ahead of time: the number of questions, the type (multiple choice, free response, etc.), and the time limit. Then create a plan for working through them. For example, if you have 30 minutes to take a 60-question test, your limit is 30 seconds per question. Spend less time on the questions you know well so that you can take more time on the difficult ones.

If you have time to take several practice tests, take the first one open book, with no time limit. Work through the questions at your own pace and make sure you fully understand them. Gradually work up to taking a test under test conditions: sit at a desk with all study materials put away and set a timer. Pace yourself to make sure you finish the test with time to spare and go back to check your answers if you have time.

After each test, check your answers. On the questions you missed, be sure you understand why you missed them. Did you misread the question (tests can use tricky wording)? Did you forget the information? Or was it something you hadn't learned? Go back and study any shaky areas that the practice tests reveal.

Taking these tests not only helps with your grade, but also aids in combating test anxiety. If you're already used to the test conditions, you're less likely to worry about it, and working through tests until you're scoring well gives you a confidence boost. Go through the practice tests until you feel comfortable, and then you can go into the test knowing that you're ready for it.

Test Tips

On test day, you should be confident, knowing that you've prepared well and are ready to answer the questions. But aside from preparation, there are several test day strategies you can employ to maximize your performance.

First, as stated before, get a good night's sleep the night before the test (and for several nights before that, if possible). Go into the test with a fresh, alert mind rather than staying up late to study.

Try not to change too much about your normal routine on the day of the test. It's important to eat a nutritious breakfast, but if you normally don't eat breakfast at all, consider eating just a protein bar. If you're a coffee drinker, go ahead and have your normal coffee. Just make sure you time it so that the caffeine doesn't wear off right in the middle of your test. Avoid sugary beverages, and drink enough water to stay hydrated but not so much that you need a restroom break 10 minutes into the test. If your test isn't first thing in the morning, consider going for a walk or doing a light workout before the test to get your blood flowing.

Allow yourself enough time to get ready, and leave for the test with plenty of time to spare so you won't have the anxiety of scrambling to arrive in time. Another reason to be early is to select a good seat. It's helpful to sit away from doors and windows, which can be distracting. Find a good seat, get out your supplies, and settle your mind before the test begins.

When the test begins, start by going over the instructions carefully, even if you already know what to expect. Make sure you avoid any careless mistakes by following the directions.

Then begin working through the questions, pacing yourself as you've practiced. If you're not sure on an answer, don't spend too much time on it, and don't let it shake your confidence. Either skip it and come back later, or eliminate as many wrong answers as possible and guess among the remaining ones. Don't dwell on these questions as you continue—put them out of your mind and focus on what lies ahead.

Be sure to read all of the answer choices, even if you're sure the first one is the right answer. Sometimes you'll find a better one if you keep reading. But don't second-guess yourself if you do immediately know the answer. Your gut instinct is usually right. Don't let test anxiety rob you of the information you know.

If you have time at the end of the test (and if the test format allows), go back and review your answers. Be cautious about changing any, since your first instinct tends to be correct, but make sure you didn't misread any of the questions or accidentally mark the wrong answer choice. Look over any you skipped and make an educated guess.

At the end, leave the test feeling confident. You've done your best, so don't waste time worrying about your performance or wishing you could change anything. Instead, celebrate the successful

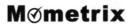

completion of this test. And finally, use this test to learn how to deal with anxiety even better next time.

> **Review Video: 5 Tips to Beat Test Anxiety**
> Visit mometrix.com/academy and enter code: 570656

Important Qualification

Not all anxiety is created equal. If your test anxiety is causing major issues in your life beyond the classroom or testing center, or if you are experiencing troubling physical symptoms related to your anxiety, it may be a sign of a serious physiological or psychological condition. If this sounds like your situation, we strongly encourage you to seek professional help.

Thank You

We at Mometrix would like to extend our heartfelt thanks to you, our friend and patron, for allowing us to play a part in your journey. It is a privilege to serve people from all walks of life who are unified in their commitment to building the best future they can for themselves.

The preparation you devote to these important testing milestones may be the most valuable educational opportunity you have for making a real difference in your life. We encourage you to put your heart into it—that feeling of succeeding, overcoming, and yes, conquering will be well worth the hours you've invested.

We want to hear your story, your struggles and your successes, and if you see any opportunities for us to improve our materials so we can help others even more effectively in the future, please share that with us as well. **The team at Mometrix would be absolutely thrilled to hear from you!** So please, send us an email (support@mometrix.com) and let's stay in touch.

> **If you'd like some additional help, check out these other resources we offer for your exam:**
> http://mometrixflashcards.com/CCTN

Additional Bonus Material

Due to our efforts to try to keep this book to a manageable length, we've created a link that will give you access to all of your additional bonus material.

Please visit https://www.mometrix.com/bonus948/cctn to access the information.